THE KINGDOM IMAGE CONSULTANT

IMAGE IS EVERYTHING

Book Four in the Identity Series

David Omondi

All rights reserved. No part of this publication may be reproduced, stored in a retrieval system, or transmitted in any form or by any means-electronic, mechanical, photocopy, recording, or any other except for brief quotations in printed or online reviews, without the prior permission of the publisher.

Unless otherwise identified, Scripture quotations are from the KING JAMES VERSION, public domain. Scriptures marked MKJV are taken from the MODERN KING JAMES VERSION (MKJV): copyright© 1962, Used by permission. Scriptures marked NKJV are taken from the NEW KING JAMES VERSION (NKJV): Copyright© 1982 by Thomas Nelson, Inc. Scripture marked NIV are taken from the NEW INTERNATIONAL VERSION (NIV): Used by permission. Scripture marked NLT are taken from the NEW LIVING TRANSLATION (NLT): Used by permission. Scripture marked ASV are taken from the AMERICAN STANDARD VERSION (ASV): Used by permission. Scripture marked AMP are taken from the AMPLIFIED BIBLE (AMP): Used by permission. Scripture marked RSV are taken from the Revised Standard Version (RSV): Used by permission.

Published by: Kingdom Fashion Revolution

© Copyright 2022 – David Omondi

info@kingdomfashion.co.ke

www.kingdomfashion.co.ke

DEDICATION

To all Christians who are waging the good fight of faith in living out their authentic and unique image and identity as they serve God and men.

So we don't look at the troubles we can see now; rather, we fix our gaze on things that cannot be seen. For the things we see now will soon be gone, but the things we cannot see will last forever. (2 Corinthians 4:18 NLT)

So we have stopped evaluating others from a human point of view. At one time we thought of Christ merely from a human point of view. How differently we know him now! (2 Corinthians 5:16 NLT)

TABLE OF CONTENTS

INTRODUCTION

The world is spiraling out of control and there's no human intervention that's able to change its trajectory. The world as we knew it pre-covid pandemic does not exist anymore. Unfortunately, the shift has been towards negative extremities.

One of the biggest casualties has been the image of people. The image has taken a beating and continues to be pounded under heavy mental and physical stress. In my home country of Kenya, data shows that one in four people is likely to experience a mental health condition. This kind of data is not unique to my country, it cuts across all nations of the world.

The image and identity of men has been fractured into small pieces and strewn all over different platforms and ideologies. The digital world promises a new universe where we can overcome the limitations and challenges of the physical world but, is it really safe. Is it possible to wholly live as a digital human as promised by the creators of the metaverse and those working hard to merge our bodies with digital technologies?

How about gender? Well, it's about how you feel. If you feel you're a woman trapped in a man's body, you can transition and become a woman and vice versa. You can identify as whatever you fancy; an animal, a gadget, nothing limits you. We live in a world where the definition of who is a woman has become a source of contention. Everything is fluid.

That's the world we live in. The standard image consultancy protocol is not sufficient to help your client or even yourself deal with the complex and dynamic factors that currently affect the image and identity of people.

One thing though, is still true; image is everything and that's why it is under a serious barrage of attacks. In the beginning, it was the image and likeness of God in man (male and female) that enabled them to have dominion over all creation in the earth. All other creation were made after their own kind but man had God as his template. Man had a divine nature that enabled him to think, speak and act like God in the earth. That image and identity carried authority and power to be fruitful, multiply, subdue, replenish and to have dominion over all principles, forces and resources, visible and invisible.

Satan knew that with man's divine image and identity intact, he had no chance to control anything in the earth. So, he devised a lie and succeeded in corrupting this image of God when he convinced Adam to disobey God. Ever since the fall of man, Satan has worked tirelessly to keep men under his dominion with corrupted and disfigured images and identity.

Thanks be to God that through the death and resurrection of Jesus Christ, the image and identity of God has been restored to all that receive Jesus Christ as Lord and Saviour, and as we continuously behold Christ as in a mirror through the Word, we're transformed into the same image from glory to glory.

Image is everything, it is what elevated man above all other creation in the beginning and it is the treasure we carry today in our earthen vessels that make us reign in this life. That image is Christ in you; when it's worked on daily, it is the antidot to the mental pandemic ravaging the world population in one way or the other.

The strategy of the enemy is to wear people down until they surrender to his control. Then he steals their joy, peace, hope, faith, love, health, soundness of mind and all the blessings that come from knowing and walking with Jesus.

The standard image consultancy playbook is no longer effective in the current world where change is happening at the speed of light on a global scale and affecting even the remotest villages. The image and identity of many people is under constant battering with not enough time to make adjustments before the next wave of change.

The good news is that there is a divine playbook that has largely been ignored by the world and one that does not fail. It has been ignored by design because the architect of the world system has no room for your divine image and identity. The standard playbook focuses on the ABCs of image consultancy which are Appearance, Behaviour and Communication with a recent addition of Digital Presence and Emotional Intelligence to make it ABCDE.

However, as you will find out in this book, the ABCDE are the secondary aspects of image and identity and by those alone, you will not surmount the challenges you or your client will face. In this book you'll find out the Kingdom definitions and standards and laws that govern image consultancy with relevant Bible examples and much more. It is time to offer Kingdom solution to the image crisis that plagues the world.

For God, who said, "Let there be light in the darkness," has made this light shine in our hearts so we could know the glory of God that is seen in the face of Jesus Christ. (2 Corinthians 4:6 NLT)

1. ONLY NAKED MEN DIE

There had never been such kind of long silence in the camp as it was that morning. All the children of Israel from the oldest to the youngest stood outside their tents with their eyes glued to the side of the mountain as if watching a movie from the big screen in a cinema hall.

Everyone knew exactly what was going down because an announcement had been made that shocked everyone. They couldn't believe what was unfolding before their eyes. God had announced that Aaron the high priest's time to die had come and it was to happen publicly before everyone.

The back story to this present scenario happened in Kadesh where the people rebelled against Moses and Aaron and they complained against God. They had journeyed and came into the desert of Zin and abode at a place called Kadesh. It was a harsh environment and there was no water to drink. It was also the place where Miriam died and was buried.

With no water and the extreme barrenness of the desert condition, the people forgot that the God who was leading them knew no impossibilities. They forgot the miracle of the parting of the red sea. They forgot that God had previously provided for them water out of a rock. They became grumpy and agitated and murmured against Moses, Aaron and God. Moses and Aaron then went to enquire from God about the solution and God gave instructions on what to do.

Moses came back and gathered the people. He was angry because of their grumblings and while addressing them, he did not obey God's command to speak to the rock but instead hit the rock twice. Water came out and the people drank but God was not pleased with Moses and Aaron and it was there that God told them they would not lead the people into the promised land.

The people afterwards journeyed from Kadesh and after a long time, they came to mount Hor and it was here that Aaron's journey was to end.

And the LORD spake unto Moses and Aaron in mount Hor, by the coast of the land of Edom, saying, Aaron shall be gathered unto his people: for he shall not enter into the land which I have given unto the children of Israel, because ye rebelled against my word at the water of Meribah. (Numbers 20: 23-24)

God told Moses to take Aaron and Eleazar his son and bring them up the mountain and strip Aaron of his high priest's garments and put them upon Eleazar his son. This scene is what was unfolding before the presence of all the children of Israel.

Moses did as God had commanded; they went up the mountain and he stripped Aaron of his garments and put them upon Eleazar and as soon as he finished, Aaron died there in the top of the mountain in the sight of all the congregation of Israel (Numbers 20: 27-29).

As long as Aaron wore the priestly garments, he could not die but immediately he removed them, he was found naked and he died. There's something that death respects, your clothing. Death cannot touch a clothed man. If people knew that their clothing was that important, they wouldn't be casual about it. Only naked men die and this tragedy has befallen many Christians today. There are many believers who are walking around naked and they have become an easy pick for Satan's attacks.

Dressing is first spiritual before it is physical. The spiritual dressing is more consequential than physical dressing. Aaron's priestly garments represented a spiritual mantle that was upon his life. It was more relevant and consequential in the spiritual realm than in the physical realm. It represented what was happening before the heavenly throne of God. The tabernacle before which Aaron ministered was a mirror of the heavenly throne where holiness is not compromised at all.

Many people take great consideration and time to pick what to wear before stepping out of their homes but fail to take equal measures if not more about their spiritual dressing. They thus step out physically elegantly dressed but spiritually naked or half naked. In the spiritual realm, there's no disguising, as the seven sons of Sceva found out the hard way.

But put ye on the Lord Jesus Christ, and make not provision for the flesh, to fulfil the lusts thereof. (Romans 13:14)

The Bible commands that we put on the Lord Jesus Christ, some translations say "clothe yourself with the Lord Jesus Christ." Interestingly, this admonition is given to believers who are already born again and have received the Lord as their saviour. So why is there a need to put on the Lord Jesus Christ?

"Putting on" is an active verb of a continuous act of purposely and enthusiastically choosing to walk with and be like Christ in thought, speech and actions. It is not enough to be saved, salvation must lead to an active godly lifestyle that influences everything we do on a daily basis and under all circumstances. That is how we maintain a successful image and identity no matter the dynamics of life.

The whole armour of God spoken about in Ephesians chapter six is not meant to be removed at any given time, yet many believers walk around with parts missing while others have nothing on at all. The helmet of salvation, the breastplate of righteousness, the belt of truth, the shield of faith and the shoes of the preparation of the gospel of peace are not optional accessories but critical wear. In fact, the whole armour of God is Christ, having it on is to put on Christ.

Christ is our salvation (helmet) Acts 4:12, He is our righteousness (breastplate) 2 Corinthians 5:21, He is the truth (belt) John 14:6, we live by His faith (shield) Galatians 2:20 and He is also the author and finisher of our faith, Hebrews 12:2. He is the good news that brings us peace and reconciliation to God (Shoes) Romans 1:16 and Romans 10:15.

Put on the whole armour of God, that ye may be able to stand against the wiles of the devil. (Ephesians 6:11)

Satan works from the outside while God works from inside. Satan uses external situations and circumstances to distort our image and identity. He uses storms, giants, invading armies, threats, intimidation, lies and deception to get us to undress on our own through fear, unbelief, doubt and surrender.

We're living in the days where the war on God's image in men has greatly intensified on all fronts. Satan is on a rampage because he senses his days are numbered. The world is experiencing tremendous shakings and all the safety nets men had built for themselves can't hold anymore. Things are crumbling at an accelerated pace beyond ability to recover.

It is the image and likeness of God in Adam and Eve that made them to have dominion over every other creation in the earth. It is the image and likeness of God that Jesus came to restore unto us through His death and resurrection. Now, as we continuously behold Him in the Word, we're transformed into the same image from glory to glory.

The person whose image and identity in Christ is intact, lives above the situations and circumstances of the earth. Satan cannot mess up with their mind because they have heavens' perspective to life that transcends the world and time.

In order to experience sustained victory in this war, we need to be properly equipped for battle. It's impossible to win a war without proper intelligence. There are too many casualties dying in the battlefield because many believers are dressed up like civilians in their mind. It is important to understand what's at stake and what it will take to be on the winning side. No child of God should perish due to ignorance. We're the ones whom God has entrusted with the message of salvation and reconciliation that the world so desperately needs and therefore, we can't be perishing like a people without God.

We carry the treasure in earthen vessels and this treasure is what the enemy is after, to destroy. It's not about the deteriorating economies, compromised politics, corruption, ungodly sexual and health rights, pandemics, climate change, wars, famines, and the others that will come. All these are a means to an end for Satan and his human agents.

The image and identity of God in you is the target. The heavens and the earth will get old like a garment, in fact God will do away with them and create a new earth and a new heaven (Hebrews 1:10-12), but for people, it's either eternal life or eternal damnation. The divine destiny of humans is the prize and it's based on one thing only, how we live out our divine image and identity while in the world.

*For **we must all appear** before the judgment seat of Christ; that every one may receive the things done in his body, according to that he hath done, whether it be good or bad. (2 Corinthians 5:10)*

Let's look at two more examples from scriptures on how working on our spiritual image and identity can alter the destiny of not only individuals, but nations.

WHO'S BETTER DRESSED FOR BATTLE?

The children of Israel were toast before Goliath. He had sent such a shiver down their spine that every time he came out to dare them, they would scatter into hiding. The entire destiny of the nation hinged on the outcome of the battle between just two people; Goliath for Philistine and whoever would step up to the plate for Israel.

Then Goliath, a Philistine champion from Gath, came out of the Philistine ranks to face the forces of Israel. He was over nine feet tall! He wore a bronze helmet, and his bronze coat of mail weighed 125 pounds. He also wore bronze leg armor, and he carried a bronze javelin on his shoulder. The shaft of his spear was as heavy and thick as a weaver's beam, tipped with an iron spearhead that weighed 15 pounds. His armor bearer walked ahead of him carrying a shield. (1 Samuel 17:4-7 NLT)

Such was the scene for forty days each morning and evening as Goliath stepped forward to ask for someone to fight from

Israel. He was a scary figure to behold. This giant of a person was ugly huge and heavily armoured and spoke boisterously and menacingly. He was truly dressed for the job and he behaved like a real champion and his communication was authoritative, clear and direct. His image consultant had done a great job.

Goliath stood and shouted to the ranks of Israel, "Why do you come out and line up for battle? Am I not a Philistine, and are you not the servants of Saul? Choose a man and have him come down to me. If he is able to fight and kill me, we will become your subjects; but if I overcome him and kill him, you will become our subjects and serve us." Then the Philistine said, "This day I defy the armies of Israel! Give me a man and let us fight each other." On hearing the Philistine's words, Saul and all the Israelites were dismayed and terrified. (1 Samuel 17:8-11 NIV)

Then, one day, David appeared on the scene and saw and heard the demand of Goliath to the children of Israel and the promise that king Saul had given for the person who would volunteer to face and kill the giant.

David was of a different mindset than the soldiers of Israel. He understood by historical knowledge that Israel belonged to God and defying Israel is equivalent to defying God. He also had experienced great personal victories by God's help against fierce wild animals and Goliath was no different. David therefore offered himself to face Goliath even though he was not yet qualified to be part of the army. King Saul was initially hesitant about sending David against Goliath but David had a compelling testimony.

But David said to Saul, "Your servant has been keeping his father's sheep. When a lion or a bear came and carried off a sheep from the flock, I went after it, struck it and rescued the sheep from its mouth. When it turned on me, I seized it by its hair, struck it and killed it. Your servant has killed both the lion and the bear; this uncircumcised Philistine will be like one of them, because he has defied the armies of the living God. The Lord who rescued me from the paw of the lion and the paw of the bear will rescue me from the hand of this Philistine." (1 Samuel 17:34-37 NIV)

The bible passage above holds the key to David's victory over Goliath because what happened next reveals to us who between him and Goliath was truly dressed for the battle.

As a soldier going to battle you must be properly kitted for war. David was dressed like a shepherd and had a shepherd's gear of rod, sling and a small bag. King Saul offered to arm him with his armour, but when David put it on, he felt hindered by it instead of protected, so he discarded it. The lesson here is, don't seek to impress outwardly with what is not consistent with your preparation for the task at hand. You will look the part but underwhelm in performance.

Next, he showed up on the battlefield and everything looked like a ridiculous mismatch. Here was a nine foot, heavily built and dangerously armoured, battle-hardened warrior coming against a young youth with no armour, no sword and no shield.

He looked David over and saw that he was little more than a boy, glowing with health and handsome, and he despised him. He said to David, "Am I a dog, that you come at me with sticks?" And the Philistine cursed David by his gods. "Come here," he said, "and I'll give your flesh to the birds and the wild animals!" (1 Samuel 17:42-44 NIV)

Notice the bible records that Goliath cursed David by his gods. This is significant because warfare is not just physical, there are spiritual forces involved. The human warrior must invoke the name and powers of his god or God if they're expecting to win. The stronger of the deities will have the victory.

Goliath was about to experience a lesson that he was not ever to recover from. While he was physically armoured like the presidential motorcade and carried lethal weaponry equivalent to a nuclear bomb against David's little round stones, spiritually, he was found naked. And that is what made all the difference in this battle.

Hear David's response to his threats and demeaning words.

David said to the Philistine, "You come against me with sword and spear and javelin, but I come against you in the name of the Lord Almighty, the God of the armies of Israel, whom you have defied. This day the Lord will deliver you into my hands, and I'll strike you down and cut off your head.

This very day I will give the carcasses of the Philistine army to the birds and the wild animals, and the whole world will know that there is a God in Israel. All those gathered here will know that it is not by sword or spear that the Lord saves; for the battle is the Lord's, and he will give all of you into our hands." (1 Samuel 17:45-47 NIV)

That's it, Goliath died and the Philistines were defeated and plundered. The nation of Israel retained their independence and freedom. Our spiritual alignment and dressing determine how successful we will navigate life and destiny shaping moments that demand leadership, initiative, resolve, skill and courage.

In life, there are many Goliaths who will show up and demand all that you've got; your life, family, resources, health, peace, salvation, finances, hope, and everything else that may help you to progress. It's the investment we make in our divine image and identity that grants us the power to slay the giants.

THE DISGUISE THAT FAILED

King Ahab was a wicked king who bothered less about obeying God but he had a good friend in the king of Judah, Jehoshaphat by name. One day, Ahab requested the king of Judah to go into battle with him. However, Jehoshaphat requested if they could find out from God first if they will achieve victory.

King Ahab assembled four hundred prophets who prophesied to him what he wanted to hear. One by one they told him to go up into battle because God would grant him victory. However, king Jehoshaphat enquired if there was any other prophet they could enquire from.

Unfortunately for Ahab, it was Micaiah, the only prophet who really heard right from God. Micaiah then offers insight into events that transpired in the spirit realm about the lying spirit that was working through the four hundred prophets and the disaster that awaited Ahab in the battlefield.

Ahab disregards Micaiah's advice and proceeds into battle albeit with a strategy to fool the enemy.

So King Ahab of Israel and King Jehoshaphat of Judah led their armies against Ramoth-gilead. The king of Israel said to Jehoshaphat, "As we go into battle, I will disguise myself so no one will recognize me, but you wear your royal robes." So the king of Israel disguised himself, and they went into battle. (2 Chronicles 18:28-29 NLT)

While it was possible for Ahab to disguise himself in the natural, it was impossible for him to do so in the spirit. Initially it seemed as if it was working because, when the enemy Aramean army saw the chariot of king Jehoshaphat, they thought it was king Ahab and they pursued hard after him. King Jehoshaphat then cried out to God and God saved him from imminent death. He really should have listened to the advice of prophet Micaiah. Nevertheless, God showed him mercy because he walked in His ways.

So when the Aramean chariot commanders saw Jehoshaphat in his royal robes, they went after him. "There is the king of Israel!" they shouted. But Jehoshaphat called out, and the LORD saved him. God helped him by turning the attackers away from him. As soon as the chariot commanders realized he was not the king of Israel, they stopped chasing him. (2 Chronicles 18:31-32 NLT)

For a season, someone may get away with changes in physical appearance and mannerisms but sooner or later, their true predisposition will be revealed. Unfortunately for king Ahab, an occurrence that seemed so random sealed his fate as a consequence of his disobedience, hence spiritual nakedness.

An Aramean soldier, however, randomly shot an arrow at the Israelite troops and hit the king of Israel between the joints of his armor. "Turn the horses and get me out of here!" Ahab groaned to the driver of the chariot. "I'm badly wounded!" The battle raged all that day, and the king of Israel propped himself up in his chariot facing the Arameans. In the evening, just as the sun was setting, he died. (2 Chronicles 18:33-34 NLT)

Sara Jane Biggart, the author of the book titled, "Seeing Beyond," talks of the spiritual reality of the life of the believer. The ability to operate spiritual senses of sight, hearing, taste, smell and touch. Our ability to partner with

God as co-labourers and friends, gives us access to see what God is doing.

In an interview with Sid Roth of "It's Supernatural" TV show, Sara recounted an experience she had while walking on a street in Glasgow. All of a sudden everything went into slow motion and the atmosphere became very still. She began to see on the people walking towards her, the spiritual clothing that they were wearing such as clothes of greed, lust, hate or fear.

She then asked God the meaning of all that was transpiring. Then God opened her ears and she began to hear the sounds that were made by these spiritual clothes. The clothes were resonating different frequencies and the clothe of spirit of fear produced the highest pitch. It was not only the highest pitch but also horrible and traveled the furthest in the spirit realm than all the others.

She then delved into the question of whether demons can read peoples' mind. Well, the answer is they don't have to because we wear what we have partnered with, whether it be fear, anger, lust, or whatever else and the demons can see it and hear it as well.

Every spiritual partnership that leaves the children of God naked and exposed to demonic spirits must be broken off. Those who are not born again have no chance unless they receive salvation. When our image and identity is disfigured in the spirit, we will malfunction in life no matter our efforts to transform our outward appearance, behaviour and communication.

Jesus Christ suffered fierce and sustained attacks on His image and identity and left us great lessons on how to handle the enemy on our own terms based on the Word of God and the intelligence of the Holy Spirit. Let's find out more in the next chapter.

2. THE IMAGE WAR

THE FIERCE IMAGE CONFLICT JESUS HAD WITH MEN

One of the areas that Jesus had the greatest contention with the Pharisees and a section of the Jews was around His identity. His identity was questioned from the beginning of His ministry to the end. Even John the Baptist whom God had sent to publicly reveal the Christ doubted at some point and had to send a few of His disciples to go ask Jesus if He was indeed the Christ.

His temptation in the wilderness by the chief tempter was around the question of identity, "if you're the son of God, then…"

The identity of Jesus was thoroughly questioned and tested throughout His ministry. At one point the Jews wanted to stone Him because He claimed that He was the Son of God. They considered the claim blasphemous because to be the Son of God is to make yourself equal with God (John 10:30-33).

After some time, Jesus asked His disciples who people said that He was and then asked them who they thought He was. This He asked not because He doubted His identity, but to find out, perhaps, some seeds of doubt had been sown in them from hearing all the false accusations surrounding His identity.

Peter replied, "You are the Christ, the Son of the living God," to which Jesus replied, "flesh and blood did not reveal that to you..."

There are good lessons we can glean about identity and image from the story of Jesus and the conflict surrounding His identity.

1. **Your identity is validated by what you do and say:** The reply of Jesus to the disciples of John if He was the Christ was simple, it was based on the works that He was doing.

   Then Jesus answering said unto them, Go your way, and tell John what things ye have seen and heard; how that the blind see, the lame walk, the lepers are cleansed, the deaf hear, the dead are raised, to the poor the gospel is preached. (Luke 7:22)

   As God's children, we have received power to be witnesses of Christ by the Holy Spirit. It is God who is at work in us both to will and to do according to His pleasure. God has empowered us and availed unto us divine provision for the assignment He has given to each of us. We have received God's image and identity in Christ to enable us to live, walk and get results like Christ in the earth.

   Verily. Verily, I say unto you, He that believeth on me, the works that I do shall he do also; and greater works than these shall he do; because I go unto my Father. (John 14:12)

2. **What you do and say is determined by your purpose:** The purposeful life is confined to the narrow path. A man that is sold out to pursue God's call in their life has no plan 'B', their path is predetermined and set. Purpose controls the why, how, where and on what you spend your time and other resources.

Success in life is what you have done compared to what you were created to do, it is the fulfillment and completion of purpose. Progress is measured by assignment, not activity. God measures success based on Jeremiah 29:11 where He has set a future, a mark ahead of you that you're supposed to reach. Your purpose charts the course and brings you to the place of good success. Knowing your God given purpose is not an option, neither is it for a later date after you're done with your other projects.

Jesus at the age of twelve knew that He had to be about the Father's business and before He finished His earthly ministry, He commanded us to do business until He comes back. Outside of your purpose, your image and identity is cast in shadows of darkness with no clarity nor focus.

3. **Your purpose and identity is revealed to you by God:** You cannot discover your identity on your own without the help of God. Your life was predestined by God and that means that your purpose, the reason for your existence was predetermined before your birth and is held by God for you.

    By flesh and blood, you cannot discover nor fulfill your purpose nor reach your full potential. Living life without God is a work in futility no matter how much you accomplish in the world. The success of every person is tied to their relationship and close walk of intimacy with God. It is out of this oneness with God that mysteries of life are revealed, knowledge, understanding and wisdom is dispensed, authority and power is given, vision and mission is downloaded.

    The person who's intimate with God cannot be confused about their image, identity, purpose and mission no matter the challenges they face. This was the case with Joseph, Nehemiah, Daniel, Mordecai, Apostle Paul, Stephen and so many others. Before you were born, God already sanctified and ordained you with the assignment you're to accomplish for Him in the earth. God did not leave it up to us to guess and figure it out, all we need is ask Him to show us and direct us into its fulfillment.

He restoreth my soul: he leadeth me in the paths of righteousness for his name's sake. (Psalm 23:3)

Before I formed thee in the belly I knew thee; and before thou camest forth out of the womb I sanctified thee, and I ordained thee a prophet unto the nations. (Jeremiah 1:5)

4. **The greatest conflict you will face in life will be around your identity.** You will face tremendous resistance in your quest to live out your divine identity. Some days it will be you questioning your own identity due to the attacks and conflicts you will face. The world will exert pressure or pleasure to resist your divine advancement or lure you through comfort (deceitfulness of riches) or ignorance as well illustrated through the parable of the sower – Luke 8:4-15.

Whatever challenge you're experiencing now that's not due to sin or ignorance, it is your image and identity in Christ being questioned and challenged. If you're the son of God, why are you in...lack..., sickness..., jobless...., single..., not yet promoted..., childless..., advancing slowly than your peers..., depressed..., etc. Satan will constantly try to find occasion to attack your image and identity. The parable of the sower ends by stating that only those with an honest and good heart, having heard the

Word, keep it, and bring forth fruit with patience –
vs 15.

The Pharisees, Sadducees and the elders constantly
followed Jesus and tried to find occasion to accuse
Him or trick Him into doing a mistake that they
might find reason to harm him. Nothing was off the
table for these evil men in their quest to snuff off
the light of Jesus. Every good thing that Jesus did,
they twisted it to look like evil.

*And he taught daily in the temple, But the chief
priests and the scribes and the chief of the people
sought to destroy him, (Luke 19:47)*

*Now the chief priests, and elders, and all the council,
sought false witness against Jesus, to put him to
death; (Matthew 26:59)*

5. **The greatest fulfillment you will ever experience is
   to live your authentic, unique and divine identity
   given to you by God.** In spite of all the conflict that
   Jesus faced concerning His identity, He lived life
   under His own terms, even His death was because
   He willingly laid down His life. Every threat and
   attempt on His life that was premature failed.

   When you truly know who you're, you will live life
   with the boldness of a lion, the dexterity of an eagle,

the strength of an ox and the humility and love of the redeemed soul.

The challenges that people have with their image is beyond appearance, behaviour and communication. The ability to dig into the root cause of the image challenge is what will set you apart from your peers as an image consultant and also ensure that you provide accurate diagnosis and solution for yourself and others.

THE IMAGE CRISIS

There's an image and identity pandemic ravaging the entire planet earth. People are desperate and confused about who they are and answers are not forthcoming either. The image crisis has been carefully crafted and manufactured by agents of the kingdom of darkness in order to catch men into snares like they do for birds.

The image crisis centers around negative worldly influences on personal freedoms and liberties, family, work environment, national and geo politics, economy, sexuality and gender, religion, race, education, sports and entertainment, fashion, beauty, science, globalization, internet, technology, climate and environment, media, and many more. Ideologies and philosophies have taken hard lines and you're either on the left or on the right. The traditional family order is being destroyed and re written to conform with the lustful desires of the flesh and mind of depraved men.

All this breed an unstable and unhealthy world where men live without constraints. News headlines that come from different parts of the world are horrific to say the least. Men behaving like animals controlled by instinct only and the drive to survive at all cost. The conscience of many has been seared and have lost the ability to empathize, qualities that separate us from animals.

THE ORIGINAL IMAGE

God's original plan was His image and likeness in man. Man was to operate as the representative of God in the earth, working together in partnership to establish heaven on earth. The image of God in man gave him the divine qualities and attributes that would enable him to build heavens' civilization on the earth.

Heaven is perfect because of the persons that reside there. If God was to move to earth and men move to heaven, the opposite would take place. The earth would become like heaven and heaven would become like the earth. It is the mindset of God and His culture that make heaven to be heaven.

The original plan allowed man to think like God. It is from how a man thinks that he develops his culture and ultimately civilization. The corrupt civilization that is preeminent in the earth is a reflection of how men think.

Adam and his offspring were given the mandate and ability to turn the whole earth into an Eden. God blessed them and commanded them to be fruitful, to multiply, to replenish, to subdue and to have dominion.

THE IMAGE CORRUPTION

Satan saw how God had given man authority over the riches and glory of the earth and made man a god over all that was in it and he couldn't fathom it. He deviously crafted a plan for a hostile takeover in order to be the god of the world.

And God said, Behold, Behold, I have given you every herb bearing seed, which is upon the face of all the earth, and every tree, in the which is the fruit of a tree yielding seed; to you it shall be for meat. (Genesis 1:29)

God gave to man every plant that carries seed and every fruit tree that yields seed as food. This is critical to note because there was one tree whose fruit bore no seeds. That means that it had no ability to multiply on its own.

And out of the ground made the LORD God to grow every tree that is pleasant to the sight, and good for food; the tree of life also in the midst of the garden, and the tree of knowledge of good and evil. (Genesis 2:9)

The tree of the knowledge of good and evil belonged to Satan and since he is not a creator, his tree had seedless fruit. Satan knew that the only way to ensure that his tree could multiply was by making man to consume it. Then as man reproduces, the fruit from his tree would naturally be reproduced into all men. That is how he would gain access and control the entire earth and exercise dominion over all men.

So, he hatched up a plan to deceive and to lie and trick man into willful disobedience against God. When Adam and Eve fell for his trick and ate Satan's fruit (idea/knowledge) there was an immediate destruction of the image of God in man.

Man took on the nature and mindset of Satan. Man's connection with God was severed leading to instant spiritual death. His soul became darkened and he was now controlled by the lusts of the flesh and mind. He lost authority over the earth and Satan instituted another governing system working through the law of sin and death.

THE SEED FROM THE TREE OF THE KNOWLEDGE OF GOOD AND EVIL

Through the disobedience of man, Satan found a way to reproduce seed from the tree of the knowledge of good and evil. Every man born into the world comes seeded with the sin nature. This means that we are born into the world unawares of our divine identity and image.

Satan capitalizes on this scenario and seeks to hinder people from coming to the knowledge of the truth about their divine identity. This he has succeeded to do by creating sub cultures around certain counterfeit images and identities.

1. The Rise of Toxic Individualism and the Culture of Consumerism

The world system thrives on isolation and individualism pegged on a loose, superficial sense of community built around the need for self-preservation among people of similar ideology. This was the problem that plagued Cain in the beginning and the people who were building the tower of babel.

Cain thought that by getting rid of Abel his life would become better, he would become the sole heir of the earth. The tower of babel builders out of their desire to protect their individual interests, banded together to build a fortress. The script has not changed because it's the same seed and fruit at work in fallen men.

Satan while still serving God as Lucifer, imagined in his heart a scenario where he would be at the center of attention and be like God. His imagination bore the seed of iniquity that led to the birth of sin.

For thou hast said in thine heart, I will ascend into heaven, I will exalt my throne above the stars of God: I will sit also upon the mount of the congregation, in the sides of the north: I will ascend above the heights of the clouds; I will be like the most High. (Isaiah 14: 13-14)

This same desire is planted in men through the sin nature and men find themselves in a rat race to attain success according to the ways of the world. This self-effort to acquire wealth, fame, influence and significance has spawned evil cravings and desires that has led to untold pain and misery.

Gambling, prostitution, human trafficking, labour exploitation, war for profit, over production of goods for profit maximization, unethical marketing, legislation of unjust laws, office and boardroom wars, termination of pregnancies in order to continue enjoying the pleasures of illicit sex and many other evil things.

All these things create toxic spiritual, mental and physical environments that interfere with people's image perceptions and identity. People are forced to band together in loose groupings for survival and a false sense of belonging and security. There are all kinds of associations out there around interests, needs, fears, aspirations, social groupings, things owned (owners associations) etc.

The religion of needs has warped the priorities of men where people are willing to sell their birth rights for a bowl of soup. They seek for quick outward transformations that will increase their chances of amassing more of the world's goods and access to services and other privileges in the hope of achieving self-actualization.

This know also, that in the last days perilous times shall come. For men shall be lovers of their own selves, covetous, boasters, proud, blasphemers, disobedient to parents, unthankful, unholy, without natural affection, trucebreakers, false accusers, incontinent, fierce, despisers of those who are good, traitors, heady, highminded, lovers of pleasures more than lovers of God; Having a form of godliness, but denying the power thereof: from such turn away. (2Timothy 1-5)

Men labour to create and maintain these false image projections because the tide of worldly culture has swept the whole earth with ungodly standards. If you don't toe the line then you can easily find yourself ostracized and unable to access certain professional and social spaces.

The person whose divine image and identity has been restored through salvation does not need to enter the rat race because it is God's pleasure to give us the Kingdom. In God's Kingdom, the economy of lack, scarcity, hoarding and greed to amass wealth doesn't exist. In the Kingdom, we're the children of the King and stewards of the Kingdom's resources and agenda.

Fear not, little flock; for it is your Father's good pleasure to give you the kingdom. (Luke 12:32)

It's the Kingdom of more than enough, the exceedingly, abundantly above all, dimension. In the Kingdom, life starts with significance whereas in the world, life starts with acquiring things in order to achieve significance. These two mindsets affect image and identity perception. For Christians, transformation is achieved by the renewing of the mind so that the good, acceptable and perfect will of God may be discovered and used to express the right image and identity through speech and action.

2. Gender and Sexual Orientation Confusion

*So God created man in his own image, in the image of God created he him; **male and female** created he them. (Genesis 1:27)*

We live in a time when some university professors, medical doctors, justices of the highest courts and politicians conveniently can't define who a woman is. This, from some of the most educated men and women in the world shows you how low the society has sunk. The idea that someone's gender is determined by feelings and not biology is nothing short of deception.

No wonder there are some children who are identifying as wolves, cats, and even as gadgets. Imagine a situation where a teacher comes into a classroom and asks a student a question and the response they receive is "meow!" The teacher can't do anything because on that particular day, the student chose to identify as a cat. There was also a video doing rounds on social media where a young man and his friend were filming within premises where it's prohibited to record video. A young lady who works there approaches them and tells them they're not allowed to film in that place. The young man who accompanied the filming friend then responds to the young lady in reference to his friend, "he identifies as a camera." The lady is visibly astounded but lets them to continue recording because it's now normal to identify as anything you wish.

There was a recent story in the media of a man in one of the countries in Central America who married an alligator. Isn't that a case of animal rights abuse? How did the alligator give consent and how will the marriage be consummated? Another man still, who identifies as "fictosexual" married a hologram image of a woman but was reportedly having trouble bonding with her. All these are mental health disorders called delusion whereby a belief or an altered reality is persistently held despite evidence or agreement to the contrary.

Male and female are God's original human genders but Satan has managed to confuse men by creating new fake genders and sexual orientations. There's a strong push from the west and among certain international organizations including the United Nations and some of its agencies to legalize homosexuality and all the other confused sexual orientations and gender ideologies.

This gender and sexual orientation confusion is now actively being peddled to children through some school textbooks and children entertainment programs. Teenagers experiencing normal biological changes as they transition into youth are deliberately being confused into transgender ideology and therapies.

This tide of woke culture is enforced by governments, global media and tech companies, the entertainment and sports industries, the medical and fashion industries among others. Lines are being blurred where transgender men are allowed to compete in women sports and transgender men are incarcerated in women prisons.

The simple verdict is that it's not working. Women are beginning to realize that allowing men to compete in female sports gives the men an unfair advantage. A recent case where two women prisoners were found pregnant was attributed to a transgender man incarcerated in that prison. It's not possible to ignore biology by assuming that a person's gender is controlled by feelings. Many people who underwent surgeries to switch genders regret their decisions. Sadly though, surgeries are permanent, if a woman surgically removes her breasts, they can't grow back.

Satan lies to people that God made a mistake when He assigned them a particular gender. He conceals the concept of divine predestination and promotes the idea of self-actualization by self-discovery and effort. This virus of self that saw him kicked out of heaven has infected the thinking of men and spread like cancer.

3. Modern Day Idols

Do not make idols or set up an image or a sacred stone for yourselves, and do not place a carved stone in your land to bow down before it. I am the LORD your God. (Leviticus 26:1 NIV)

God expressly forbade the children of Israel from worshipping idols. He told them not to mingle with the other nations as their idol worshipping ways would be a snare unto them. Why did God not want the children of Israel to worship idols which were nothing more but carvings or molten images from wood, stone, silver or gold? Idols have no life in them.

Their land also is full of idols; they worship the work of their own hands, that which their own fingers have made: (Isaiah 2:8)

The worship of idols is one of the great deceptions of Satan to make men to imagine that they can create their own gods. Man was created to be in charge over the earth and all its affairs. However, man was to rule in partnership with God. The fall of man created a separation between man and God and it is this void that men seek to fill by creating idols.

However, behind idols are demons and their master Satan who crave worship from men. These demon powers manipulate and distort the image of men through divination, familiar spirits, lying spirits, spirits of lust and pride, spirits of fornication and adultery, low self-esteem or superiority complex.

What say I then? That the idol is any thing, or that which is offered in sacrifice to idols is any thing? But I say, that the things which the Gentiles sacrifice, they sacrifice to devils, and not to God: and I would not that ye should have fellowship with devils. (1 Corinthians 10: 19-20)

An idol is anything that takes center stage in your heart above God. The heart was created for only one resident and that person is God. Any other resident is a squatter and a dangerous intruder that come not for your good but as a stumbling block that diverts to destruction.

Son of man, these men have set up their idols in their heart, and put the stumbling block of their iniquity before their face: should I be enquired of at all by them? (Ezekiel 14:3)

Modern day idols may include but not limited to; academic achievements, career achievements, relationships (spouse, children, connections), beauty and body features generally, material wealth, fame, influence, knowledge, wisdom, among others.

When you find greater fulfillment in things or yourself or someone else more than in your relationship with God, then you have an idol lurking in your heart. Everyone becomes like the object of their worship and there's nothing human or human made that can satisfy the heart's longing for the divine other than God Himself.

There's no educational degree, career position, relationship connection, physical beauty or material wealth that can bring fulfillment in life or save the soul of man from sin nature. There are also situations that arise in life that if God doesn't intervene then the person involved has no way out.

There's only one God and only Him deserve our worship and adoration.

Therefore say unto the house of Israel, Thus saith the Lord GOD; Repent, and turn yourselves from your idols; and turn away your faces from all your abominations. (Ezekiel 14:6)

And what agreement hath the temple of God with idols? For ye are the temple of the living God; as God hath said, I will dwell in them, and walk in them; and I will be their God, and they shall be my people. (2 Corinthians 6:16)

The Kingdom image consultant must be aware of these idols that men worship and steer away from reinforcing the same or from helping a client to create one. Self-worship is a major problem in this age of social media where people compete to show off online for the offering basket of likes, comments and shares. This self-worship is promoted via the music and entertainment industry, film, digital games, pro-choice organizations, LGBTQ+ movement, fashion and beauty industry, among others.

4. Education Curriculum Revision

Education curriculums are being revised and re written in most parts of the world. New radical ideologies are being introduced that really have no place in the classroom. Children are being sexualized from a tender age and taught explicit stuff without parents' knowledge or consent.

Children being much more impressionable are an easy target for Satan. Confuse them while they're still young and they'll stick to it as adults. Keep the parents busy trying to earn a living and sneak on the children with worldly influence and philosophy.

The thought that parents authority over their children is being eroded by governments is against the order that God has put in place for families. Consider this case that recently happened in one of the western nation's where a teacher managed to confuse a child about their gender and the child got scheduled to undergo some medical procedures to transition gender. When the parent refused, he got arrested and arraigned in court for interfering with the rights of the child.

The world's education system has no room for God nor His Word. Parents must take great care and responsibility to ensure that their children grow in the knowledge of God and are able to discern between good and evil from a tender age. Where possible, home school your children. Realize that the school environment has changed and don't allow the enemy to influence your child's philosophy on life.

Train up a child in the way he should go: and when he is old, he will not depart from it. (Proverbs 22:6)

This scripture is primarily directed at parents, don't delegate this responsibility to a school. It is you the parent that will be answerable before God on the kind of training you gave to your child. If a child's image and identity is molded early, they'll have less challenges as adults and will be able to stand up firmly against all satanic onslaughts.

Joash was seven years when he began his reign as king in Jerusalem and he reigned for forty years. The testimony that he received from God was, he did what was right before the LORD. The secret to his success was the guidance he received from Jehoiada the priest who offered wise counsel from the Word of God.

All scripture is given by inspiration of God, and is profitable for doctrine, for reproof, for correction, for instruction in righteousness: That the man of God may be perfect, thoroughly furnished unto all good works. (2 Timothy 3:16-17)

The Word of God is the image perfecter in men that Satan has managed to remove from the education system and replaced it with false ideologies and philosophies that mutilate the image and identity of God right from kindergarten to the universities. Nothing good happens by chance, parents must take charge of their children's education, especially the knowledge of God's Word and His Kingdom.

5. Digital Fragmentation of Image

The image of the modern-day person is split into smaller pieces and spread across different digital platforms. This fragmentation continues to grow in diversity and complexity with each passing day. The myriad social media platforms, mobile Apps and websites, each having their own ecosystem demands different postures from the same person.

The rise of digital identity integration, surveillance technology, artificial intelligence and internet of things is promising to merge our biology with technology into one seamless ecosystem. The metaverse, for example, promises an entire immersive and enduring wholly digital based life experience.

The metaverse promises that anyone can overcome the limitation of the physical body in it. You can have the body of your dream, you can be any gender you want, dress like a king and travel the world through your avatar. This counterfeit universe has the potential to throw many into deception about the true nature of the human being.

The metaverse is a programmed world created by men and every experience in it, is deliberately intended to illicit a certain reaction and mindset from the users. To trust man to create a perfect world without God, is to eat the forbidden fruit all over again and expect a different result.

The fake image created in the metaverse called the avatar is the counterfeit of the spirit of a man. All its capabilities are built on digital illusion with no eternal value but rather, negative consequences in this life and judgement at the end of the age.

All these technological developments are happening at break neck speed and are being tried out and implemented in various parts of the world. Maintaining the digital image of a person is currently a challenge and the additional developments especially around digital IDs will pose new problem areas.

The fragmented image is a challenge that the Kingdom image consultant should be aware of and find solutions for their clients struggling to handle their online presence on the various digital platforms. The example we read about of a man who married a hologram is a perfect example of the deception of illusion created by digital platforms where people can't tell reality from fiction.

6. Deliberate Creation of Crisis Situations to Force Image and Identity Change

*How art thou fallen from heaven, O Lucifer, son of the morning! How art thou cut down to the ground, which **didst weaken the nations!** (Isaiah 14: 12)*

The events of the year 2020 have proven that indeed we're in the last days. Who would have imagined that it was possible to shut down the whole world? Who would have imagined the lockdowns and restrictions that were imposed by governments were possible to that scale? The suffering and the deaths experienced were unlike anything the world has experienced in recent times.

It reminds me of the story of Esther, Mordecai and Haman in the Bible. Haman became furious at Mordecai because he refused to bow the knee in obeisance. Haman began looking for a way to harm Mordecai and, in the process discovered that he was a Jew. He realized that what Mordecai refused to do was part of the culture of an entire people.

He then changed his mind to hatch a plot on how to annihilate the entire Jewish population in the empire. He came up with an excuse that the Jews were not subject to the king and therefore the king should issue a decree to destroy all of them.

And Haman said unto king Ahasuerus, there is a certain people scattered abroad and dispersed among the people in all the provinces of thy kingdom; and their laws are diverse from all people; neither keep they the king's laws: therefore it is not for the king's profit to suffer them. If it please the king, let it be written that they may be destroyed: and I will pay ten thousand talents of silver to the hands of those that have the charge of the business, to bring it into the king's treasuries. (Esther 3:8-9)

You know the rest of the story. The point is, Satan stirs up evil men who have access to governments or large powerful organizations and corporates and instigate creation of laws, regulations and policies that can destroy entire nations, economies, impose restrictions on religious beliefs, start wars and impose a new order in society. These forced resets leave citizens powerless and economically deprived.

Meanwhile, those in power end up with more power and the gap between the rich and poor grow like the distance between the Atlantic coast of Africa and the Atlantic coast of the Americas.

When events that are beyond the control of people take place, their hope gets shattered, their joy diminished and their spirit is crashed. These, then become an easy target to manipulate and control. Their image is buried and though they're still alive, they just go through the motions of life with no sense of purpose or value. That's why the vocabulary of struggle and survival has replaced the vocabulary of hope and possibilities of the period just before the Covid pandemic hit.

This deliberate oppression that the instigators have learnt to conveniently find excuse for since time immemorial continues to play out because of greed. Behind it all is Satan exploiting the sinful nature in fallen man. Only those who have a strong concept of divine identity and image can muster the faith required to overcome this kind of satanic onslaught.

Another example is found in the Bible when envious government officials hatched a devious plan to stop Daniel from being promoted to be the leader over them. They could not find any mistake on Daniel, so they suggested the creation of a new law that would make it impossible for Daniel to connect with the source of his image and identity – the source of his wisdom, authority and power - God.

Then the presidents and princes sought to find occasion against Daniel concerning the kingdom; but they could find none occasion nor fault; forasmuch as he was faithful, neither was there any error or fault found in him. Then said these men, We shall not find any occasion against this Daniel, except we find it against him concerning the law of his God. (Daniel 6:4-5)

When unjust laws, rules, mandates, policies and regulations are passed that end up fundamentally undermining the ability of people to be productive and to enjoy God-given liberties, the cascading effects affect every sphere of life.

Mental illness cases and depression soar, domestic violence, suicides, crime, divorce, fear, anger, envy, jealousy, stinginess and poverty increase. These things destabilize, mar, diminish and ultimately destroy the image and identity of people. Plans and career paths are thrown into disarray, the work environment becomes unstable and unpredictable.

God will ultimately punish these evil men, but, in the meantime, it's important to know these root causes of image challenges so that the Kingdom image consultant can provide accurate diagnosis and remedy.

Woe to those who make unjust laws, to those who issue oppressive decrees, to deprive the poor of their rights and withhold justice from the oppressed of my people, making widows their prey and robbing the fatherless. What will you do on the day of reckoning, when disaster comes from afar?

To whom will you run for help? Where will you leave your riches? (Isaiah 10: 1-3)

Behind the human agents is Satan who incites them the way he did at one time to cause king David to number the people instead of trusting in God to be his shield. Look at how Satan boasts in the scripture below about his destruction and plundering of nations.

For he says: "'By the strength of my hand I have done this, and by my wisdom, because I have understanding. I removed the boundaries of nations, I plundered their treasures; like a mighty one I subdued their kings. As one reaches into a nest, so my hand reached for the wealth of the nations; as people gather abandoned eggs, so I gathered all the countries; not one flapped a wing, or opened its mouth to chirp.'" (Isaiah 10:13-14 NIV)

3. THE KINGDOM ASSIGNMENT OF THE IMAGE CONSULTANT

As in all assignments given by God to His children to fulfill, we must be able to articulate the need of God that we're supposed to meet. Without understanding God's need, we risk being successful in the wrong assignment. That's why for the Kingdom image consultant, your learning must go beyond the standard ABCs. Let's delve in and find out what makes a successful image consultant according to the Kingdom of God.

THE SAMARITAN WOMAN

There's only one perfect image and that image is the desire of all men whether they know it or not. That image is Christ. The Kingdom image consultant's ultimate goal is to help their client through wisdom to become more Christlike.

The ability of the consultant to analyze the real problem and to prescribe the right Kingdom solution is what will determine the level of success achieved. The example of Jesus and the Samaritan woman is perfect. Jesus by perception knew exactly what the woman's problem was but He needed the cooperation of the woman and it was His approach that made all the difference.

In the fulness of time Christ came as God had promised in Genesis chapter three. He came to restore the Kingdom and also the image of God that got marred by sin. The Samaritan woman was a troubled lady. She was likely not wanted by the other women in town because she was probably a home wrecker.

I have heard a preacher say that it was due to her bad reputation that she went to the well at noon all by herself. The customary practice was that women went to the well early in the morning and often in the company of other women. This particular woman had a tainted image and was in desperate need for transformation.

Any change in appearance, behaviour and communication would not have worked for her, it would only have raised more suspicion within the community. For example, is she upgrading herself to steal more husbands? She needed a transformation that no image consultant using only the standard principles of image consultancy would have given her. When someone has been in five marriages that failed and is now on the sixth with somebody else's husband, the issues at hand are deeper and a spiritual landmine.

How would you start to help such a person? Well, Jesus began from a common ground that was not so common. The only common link was water but it wasn't common either because Jesus was a Jew and the woman was a Samaritan. These two groups of people did not relate and the woman found it strange for a Jew to ask a Samaritan for water.

There cometh a woman of Samaria to draw water: Jesus saith unto her, Give me to drink. (John 4:7)

The natural situation and need of the woman was water but Jesus only used the natural water as a conversation starter to lead towards the real and spiritual need of the woman and the solution.

Then saith the woman of Samaria unto him, How is it that thou, being a Jew, askest drink of me, which am a woman of Samaria? For the Jews have no dealings with the Samaritans. Jesus answered and said unto her, If thou knewest the gift of God, and who it is that saith to thee, Give me to drink; thou wouldest have asked of him, and he would have given thee living water. (John 4: 9-10)

The water in the well is like the clothes, accessories and make-up we wear to project our physical appearance. The image we create with clothes and accessories is temporary and we have to change it every day the same way we drink water every day to quench our thirst. The inward image is the real deal that if we fix, then we become wholesome and helps us to align with God's purpose inside and out.

Jesus mentioned a different kind of water which piqued the interest of the woman because she had never heard of water that quenches thirst once for good. The living waters sounded attractive because she would never have to come to the well again at odd hours to avoid the accusing looks of the other women. Her history bothered her but she had no way of altering the facts, they were stuck with her like a tick on the neck of a cow.

She asked Jesus to give her the living waters to meet her daily and temporary need of natural water. This would help her to keep away from the people who kept reminding her of her failures and shame. But Jesus was interested in fixing her life for good, not through an escape strategy but a transformation strategy. Many people seek the services of an image consultant in order to take care of a certain crossroad of life, scale a threshold or overcome a crisis. However, what they really need is something that brings wholesomeness and cohesion in their entire being and life, not just for the present season or phase in life but for life into eternity.

Jesus answered and said unto her, Whosoever drinketh of this water shall thirst again: But whosoever drinketh of the water that I shall give him shall never thirst; but the water that I shall give him shall be in him a well of water springing up into everlasting life. (John 4: 13-14)

You see, only the image of God in us has the ability to lift us up above our past and current failures and set us up for victory and fulfillment in life. Wardrobe change, mastering all kinds of etiquette and improving our communication skills only, is like applying makeup to a corpse. Someone might think that the corpse example is extreme but think about it, Jesus said that without Him, we can do nothing - John 15-5. That means that without Christ, we're as good as dead. The Samaritan woman had no chance in this life to redeem her image and reputation, except for Jesus who stepped in with a heavenly perspective and solution.

As they continued their conversation, Jesus took it a notch higher to bring her to the place where she would recognize and accept the solution that would sort her image and reputation problem. Jesus using the gift of discernment, knew information concerning her private life. When the woman heard about her failed relationships and other secrets of her life, she perceived in her heart that she was in the presence of a prophet and the story takes a different turn into the topic of who and where to worship.

Who you worship determines your image and identity. Everyone resembles the deity that they worship because whoever or whatever you worship becomes your source. The Samaritan woman's image and identity would not have been restored if her relationship with the true God was not first restored. Worship is the bridge that allows interaction with the divine and connects the transforming power of the Word and Spirit of God to work in us, shaping and molding us into Christlikeness.

But the hour cometh, and now is, when the true worshippers shall worship the Father in spirit and in truth: for the Father seeketh such to worship him. God is a Spirit: and they that worship him must worship him in spirit and in truth. (John 4:23-24)

Our image and identity is a spiritual work first before it becomes a mind and body work. Transformation that bears fruit that abides, start with our spiritual connection and fellowship with God. Once this is established, working on the mind and body becomes easy, rejuvenating, purposeful and impactful.

This whole conversation was a build up to the point where Jesus revealed Himself to the woman that indeed He was the Christ. The woman not only believed in Him but she ran back into town and summoned everyone to come listen to someone who knew all her life story and one who provided the solution to all her problems and predicaments. That woman and that city was never the same again.

And many of the Samaritans of that city believed on him for the saying of the woman, which testified, He told me all that ever I did. So when the Samaritans were come unto him, they besought him that he would tarry with them: and he abode there two days. And many more believed because of his own word; And said unto the woman, Now we believe, not because of thy saying: for we have heard him ourselves, and know that this is indeed the Christ, the Saviour of the world. (John 4:39-42)

The final testimony of the Samaritans is that they believed that Jesus was the Christ, the Saviour of the world. That is the end goal of the Kingdom image consultant, to bring their client to the place where Christ is solely and completely exalted as Lord and Saviour and the template upon which their image and identity is built and daily renewed by the Word of God.

RESTORING THE IMAGE

As we had established earlier, the need for an image consultant often come up during seasons of change, when someone is at a crossroad, or a threshold, or a time of crisis. Generally, people who engage an image consultant struggle with clothing choices and coordination. They don't know what to wear and where.

They're uncomfortable and unsure on the way they look and don't know where to start. They're not aware of what kind of image they're projecting, however, they know they're not achieving their life goals. The established need indicates that they're ready to embark on a path of a positive personal and professional development.

An image consultant is the right choice to help them in this journey of self-awareness through powerful self-presentation. However, as we have learnt from the story of the Samaritan woman, there's usually more than can be revealed using the standard client discovery session.

The crossroads, thresholds and the predicaments of life stem from the spiritual dimension and solutions have to stem from there first before tackling the physical look, mannerisms and effective communication. All the problems of humankind can be traced back to the fall of Adam and Eve. The solution can also be traced back to the promise and fulfillment of the remedy that God provided.

Christ is the perfect image and every man receives restoration through salvation. Without salvation, it doesn't matter how elegantly dressed and how polished their manners is, that person's standing (righteousness) is like filthy rags (Isaiah 64:6). Therefore, the assignment of the Kingdom image consultant is to first, skillfully guide their client to salvation and if already born again, plug the knowledge gap of the client in regards to their divine image and identity. This is the first and most critical step.

The Word of God is also the best guide book on appearance, behaviour and communication, but all these are only beneficial to the person who bears the image of Christ. Without the image of Christ, all remedies lack eternal value and every investment will ultimately fall short because all the activities of life must lead towards the fulfillment of God's purpose for the individual person. There's no purpose outside of Christ.

If all you succeed to do as a Kingdom image consultant is to help your client to improve their appearance, behaviour and communication, then you would have failed in your Kingdom assignment. Many evil people, conmen, fraudsters, murderers, rapists, and their ilk have learnt and mastered the art of appearance, etiquette and communication and have way led many to grievous injuries and loss of life, money, property and relationships.

There has to be something more that you offer as a Kingdom image consultant, otherwise, you may have as a client the latest swindler in town and you won't know it. The image of Christ is tied to your client's preordained purpose and assignment. Your consultancy work is a collaboration between you and the Holy Spirit to help align your client to the predestined image in God's book.

THE IMAGE BOOK

There's an image book in heaven for every person on earth. That image book is detailed to the minutest aspects of a person. This is what Jeremiah testified to when he said that God knew him before he was formed in his mother's womb (Jeremiah 1:5). Other scriptures also testify to the detailed record that God keeps of every individual.

Thine eyes did see my substance, yet being unperfect; and in thy book all my members were written, which in continuance were fashioned, when as yet there was none of them. (Psalms 139:16)

But the very hairs of your head are all numbered. (Matthew 10:30)

This image book is the reference point from which you must, with the help of the Holy Spirit, read the original specifications that God ordained for your client. This is exactly what Jesus did with the Samaritan woman.

The image of Christ is the template from which the unique identity and personality of every person is founded and built. The Kingdom image consultant works with their client to bring them to the place where they desire and choose to fulfill the scriptures in the book of Romans 12:1-2

Therefore, I urge you, brothers and sisters, in view of God's mercy, to offer your bodies as a living sacrifice, holy and pleasing to God – this is your true and proper worship. Do not conform to the pattern of this world, but be transformed by the renewing of your mind. Then you will be able to test and approve what God's will is – his good, pleasing and perfect will. (Romans 12:1-2 NIV)

In this short passage of scripture is captured the success formula for your prospective client. The body as we will shortly find out its purpose in detail, is to be offered up as a living sacrifice to God. That confines and defines the context under which the body is to operate. The scripture provides the access and limitations under which the body is required to function. This include looking into what's put in and on the body.

Renewing the mind to know the good, pleasing and perfect will of God is the place where the right direction is pointed out for your client at life's crossroad. Every threshold they come to will turn into a stepping stone and if in a crisis situation, then salvation will be secured. What better solution can there be than to know the will of God for your life?

THE PURPOSE OF THE BODY

A large percentage of the work of an image consultant involves the change of a client's physical appearance. The goal might be to achieve life goals but one of the steps is to communicate to the mind that the journey to better things has begun by working on appearance. What we see has the capacity to trigger a mental shift into a new image and hope of possibilities in life. Whereas real change and transformation must start from the inside, we can pull triggers from the outward and use them as cues for the mind.

The body is what gives us the license to operate on the earth. It is therefore vital that we take good care of it so that it can serve us optimally to aid us in accomplishing God's purpose. When the body is sick, injured or stressed, our capacity to work is hampered or slowed down and if it dies, then we can do no more on the earth.

For the most part though, the body is subjected to abuse by both Christians and non-Christians. It is subjected to unnecessary stress, toxic foods, dangerous chemicals, unnatural activities and exposed to evil forces that distort, disfigure and cause it to malfunction.

God in His Word provides specific use for the body, it's purpose and the kind of environment and conditions under which it's supposed to operate in. It is our responsibility to know, understand and use the body under these conditions to avoid the sufferings experienced by many through sickness, accidents, demonic afflictions and consequences of other wrong use.

1. THE TEMPLE OF GOD

What? Know ye not that your body is the temple of the Holy Ghost which is in you, which ye have of God, and ye are not your own? (1 Corinthians 6:19)

In order to understand the meaning of the scripture above, we have to look into what a temple is. As per the Old Testament account, the temple was the place where men worshipped God and offered sacrifices. The temple also hosted the presence of God. The person who ministered in the temple was called a priest.

The worship ordinance was determined by God Himself and the priests had to strictly follow the set protocols. As in all other religions, the deity determines the worship rituals done in the respective temples or place of worship. For example, you cannot perform Hindu worship rituals in the Muslim Mosque and vice versa.

In the New Testament, the born-again believer's body is the temple and the person is the priest in charge of offering sacrifices. This understanding is critical because the temple should not be defiled but kept as per the requirements of God. The body of the believer should be offered as a living sacrifice, holy and acceptable to God (Romans 12:1).

2. AN INSTRUMENT OF RIGHTEOUSNESS

The body of the believer is a tool that he or she uses to execute acts of righteousness in alignment with God's will and purpose for their lives. The body must be trained in righteousness until it gets into an automatic rhythm (1 Corinthians 9:27). Life on earth is lived through the body. All the good or bad that we experience or witness on the earth are results of speech and actions delivered through the body.

Therefore do not let sin reign in your mortal body so that you obey its evil desires. Do not offer any part of yourself to sin as an instrument of wickedness, but rather offer yourselves to God as those who have been brought from death to life; and offer every part of yourself to him as an instrument of righteousness. (Romans 6:12-13 NIV)

God strongly advises His children in the scripture above to avoid using their bodies to commit acts of wickedness. Rather, we're to submit our bodies under God's authority because we shall be judged or rewarded according to what we did or did not do through the body (2 Corinthians 5:10). The life to come will be determined by how we lived our lives through our bodies. How profound is that and knowing that there's nothing that is hidden before God, how ought we to conduct our affairs in public and private?

Sexual sins are nowadays celebrated and openly promoted in all forms of media. Yet, it's one of those sins that God says has a direct consequence on the body of the person involved. Many people seem to be oblivious to the damage that is done to the body as a result of sexual sins.

The unnatural sexual acts of sodomy promoted as alternative lifestyle, the legalization of abortion, the silent venom of sexually transmitted diseases, the psychological pain and trauma of adultery and fornication, the destroyed marriages, families and relationships. Sexual sins are a Tsunami of evil and misery.

Flee fornication. Every sin that a man doeth is without the body; but he that committeth fornication sinneth against his own body. (1 Corinthians 6:18)

For if you live according to the flesh, you will die; but if by the Spirit you put to death the misdeeds of the body, you will live. (Romans 8:13 NIV)

Many people have messed up their reputation and careers because of inability to master the lustful desires of the body. Appetites must be brought under strict discipline before they overwhelm and take over control of our lives through the body. Some people are addicted to good things such as food, clothes, social media, physical fitness, work, etc. Wisdom is to strike a healthy balance so that all facets of life are well taken care of in terms of time and resource allocation in accordance with God's will and righteousness.

All things are lawful unto me, but all things are not expedient: all things are lawful for me, but I will not be brought under the power of any. Meats for the belly, and the belly for meats: but God shall destroy both it and them. Now the body is not for fornication, but for the Lord; and the Lord for the body. (1 Corinthians 6:12-13)

3. PART OF CHRIST

Our individual bodies are the building blocks of the body of Christ. As you have experienced many times, when you hurt the tiniest part of your body, your whole body feels it and reacts. The pain impacts the whole body. The opposite is also true, when you're enjoying your favourite delicacy, your whole body relaxes and becomes at ease as you savour every mouthful.

Sometimes, we may feel like we're an insignificant part in the body of Christ but nothing could be further from the truth. Consider this example, when you're walking outside on your way to work or an event and a bird decides to desecrate on your jacket, shirt or blouse, your entire outfit loses its appeal and the scramble to find a way to change or clean up begins. A small unwanted spot on your attire spoils the entire look.

As individuals, we're a small part of the body of Christ, yet, when we get out of sync with the rest of the body, we stick out like a sore thumb or that bird poop on the blouse or shirt. We therefore ought to conduct our affairs in a way that does not bring disrepute to the name of Christ or cause Him to be crucified again.

Do you not know that your bodies are members of Christ Himself? Shall I then take the members of Christ and unite them with a prostitute? Never! (1 Corinthians 6:15 NIV)

4. OWNED BY GOD

People are very defensive about their personal rights and freedoms and rightly so. We live in a world where evil men are constantly scheming on how to dominate our bodies and turn them into their slaves. God did not give anybody dominion over any other human being. The mandate was to dominate everything else on the earth except human beings (Genesis 1:26-28).

However, man was not created to live independent of God. Man without God is dead and that is exactly what happened when Adam disobeyed God. The fall of man brought us under the heavy yoke of slavery to Satan, sin and death. Thankfully, Jesus paid the price for our redemption and now we have the opportunity to be reconciled back to God.

Christ purchased us with His own blood from the slave market of sin and now we no longer live for ourselves but for Him who redeemed us. Our freedom is not for doing whatever we want with our bodies, but to serve God within the loving framework of the Father's royal family as kings and priests, co-working in the family business of reconciling the world.

For ye are bought with a price: therefore glorify God in your body, and in your spirit, which are God's (1 Corinthians 6:20).

5.   USED FOR SERVING GOD AND MAN

Men and women are born into the world to serve the purpose of God as we serve each other with our gifts and talents. There's no fulfillment in living life just for yourself, that's why amassing things is not the path to happiness as many come to discover. We can learn from Solomon as he records his findings in several places in the book of Ecclesiastes. Chasing after things for the sake of owning them can be chasing after vanity.

For, brethren, ye have been called unto liberty; only use not liberty for an occasion to the flesh, but by love serve one another. (Galatians 5:13)

For the kingdom of God is not a matter of eating and drinking, but of righteousness, peace and joy in the Holy Spirit, because anyone who serves Christ in this way is pleasing to God and receives human approval. (Romans 14:17-18 NIV)

REDEFINING TERMS

The original image consultancy playbook has the authentic definition of terms and the service delivery charter. You must master image consultancy from the original playbook – the Bible – if you're going to be relevant and be on the A-list of super successful image consultants in this age of the "new normal," also known as, gross darkness. It's no longer enough to master the art of communication; the game changer is mastering both the art and the spirit of communication.

The following elements of image consultancy have been redefined to align with the Kingdom concept of the same:

- Image
- Consultant
- Consultancy
- Appearance
- Behaviour
- Communication
- Digital Presence
- Emotional balance/intelligence

Let's look into their Kingdom meaning one by one.

IMAGE: This is the original unique personality that God gives to each person built upon the template of Christ. This image contains an individual's gifts, talents, physical attributes and the unique purpose they're called to fulfill for God on the earth.

The fulness of a person's image is revealed to them as their unique identity by the Holy Spirit. As a person receives salvation and continues to walk with God on their predestined path of righteousness, the more they are able to know, express, enjoy and have good success in their life.

For those God foreknew he also predestined to be conformed to the image of his Son, that he might be the firstborn among many brothers and sisters. (Romans 8:29 NIV)

But the path of the just is as the shining light, that shineth more and more unto the perfect day. (Proverbs 4:18)

CONSULTANT: This is a Kingdom technician called to co-labour with God in helping a person to gain understanding and be rightly positioned, to better live out their divine image and identity. The Kingdom technician understands the image principles (discussed in the next chapter) necessary to redirect a person to their unique path of righteousness.

The lips of the righteous feed many: but fools die for want of wisdom. (Proverbs 10:21)

Wisdom strengtheneth the wise more than ten mighty men which are in the city. (Ecclesiastes 7:19)

Who is as the wise man? And who knoweth the interpretation of a thing? A man's wisdom maketh his face to shine, and the boldness of his face shall be changed. (Ecclesiastes 8:1)

CONSULTANCY: The professional presentation and delivery of services that help people to align themselves with Christ and rightly articulate their unique divine identity in order to fulfill purpose. This work of consultancy is carried out according to the Kingdom blueprint as outlined in the Word of God.

If the iron be blunt, and he do not whet the edge, then must he put to more strength: but wisdom is profitable to direct. (Ecclesiastes 10:10)

Happy is the man that findeth wisdom, and the man that getteth understanding. (Proverbs 3:13)

APPEARANCE: This is the outward presentation of a person as informed by an internal posture of righteousness and a mind centered on Christ and commitment to do the will of God. Appearance starts from the spirit of the man, then the soul and finally find expression through the body in the form of speech and actions.

Herein is our love made perfect, that we may have boldness in the day of judgment: because as he is, so are we in this world. (1 John 4:17)

For you were once darkness, but now you are light in the Lord. Live as children of light. (for the fruit of the light consists in all goodness, righteousness and truth). (Ephesians 5:8-9)

Jesus Christ is clothed in a garment of light and He is our light and the light of the world (John 1:4). We are children of light and are clothed in light because as He is, so are we. Light represents divine knowledge and this knowledge is truth, righteousness, holiness, purity, integrity, love, discretion, among other godly attributes.

Dressing, grooming and how you exercise yourself ought to be as a result of the influence of godly attributes. Righteousness is not a choice for the believer, it is the way of life. Physical appearance is a reflection of the internal appearance (knowledge), get it right internally and you'll get it right outwardly.

For God, who commanded the light to shine out of darkness, hath shined in our hearts, to give the light of the knowledge of the glory of God in the face of Jesus Christ. (2 Corinthians 4:6)

BEHAVIOUR: This is how we react and express how we feel in response to spiritual, soulical and physical impulses emanating from our surrounding environment. The reaction or expression of how we feel is captured and conveyed by the five physical senses of sight, sound, touch, smell and taste.

Whereas behaviour is expressed through the physical senses, it is either a product of the fruit of the Spirit or of the flesh with its corrupt desires. You cannot go wrong with the fruit of the Spirit; it is perfect behaviour because it is divinely sourced. It is the gold standard for character against which we measure ourselves.

The fruit of the Spirit interprets the impulses we receive from the environment through the physical senses and then recommends the appropriate response. For example, how to handle an angry outburst from an agitated customer who is misinformed. Do you lash back, keep quiet, apologize, explain? What do you do first and then what follows?

But the fruit of the Spirit is love, joy, peace, longsuffering, gentleness, goodness, faith, meekness, temperance: against such there is no law. (Galatians 5:22)

Since it is a fruit, it means that there's process involved in growing it. As someone grows in the fruit of the Spirit, the less of the following negative behaviour shall be exhibited until they're no more: anxiety, anger, jealousy, malice, lying, depression, worry, fear, timidity and the many others listed in the book of Galatians chapter five.

Work to grow in the fruit of the Spirit through renewing the mind and exercising yourself in godliness, which is profitable in all things (1 Timothy 4:8). All etiquette and protocol that you will need to observe in professional, social, public and private engagements are covered by the fruit of the Spirit.

COMMUNICATION: This is the ability to put forth your ideas and thoughts in an easy-to-understand way. The essence of good communication is truth and love. Where these act as the basis for communication, corruption will not be found.

Instead, speaking the truth in love, we will grow to become in every respect the mature body of him who is the head, that is Christ. (Ephesians 4:15 NIV)

Truth and love enable you to be graceful in your communication, a quality that the world cannot have because grace is a divine quality. Graceful communication allows you to interact with anyone without feeling superior or inferior but at ease, confident and respectful with your juniors, peers and seniors.

Let your conversation be always full of grace, seasoned with salt, so that you may know how to answer everyone. (Colossians 4:6 NIV)

Truth and love enable you to communicate accurately and consistently in both verbal and non-verbal communication. We all have experienced at some point a situation where what was being voiced and the communication from the body was not matching. Communication is often the deal maker or breaker of many relationships and business transactions.

For in many things we offend all. If any man offend not in word, the same is a perfect man, and able also to bridle the whole body. (James 3:2)

Communication also entails understanding how to structure information using different mediums, choice of words and the role of listener and receiver. Should you be responding or reacting to be successful in your communication? When communication is concise, precise, sincere and timely, no room will be created for misunderstanding. All these aspects are important considerations in mastering the art and spirit of communication.

DIGITAL PRESENCE: This is your capability to manage and portray a consistent personal outlook on all virtual platforms where your image is represented. Your digital accounts give you a platform to introduce, position and serve your image to the world.

Through digital platforms, someone can access global opportunities for work, business, friendship, collaboration, current news and trends among others. Digital platforms give you access to send and receive vital communication in real time.

The digital world is a mirror but far inferior reflection of the spirit realm. Internet communication allows someone to experience a sort of omni presence effect where communication can happen live on a global scale. Whereas all digital platforms have serious security and privacy issues, we use them because they provide an easy entry point and platform to interact and influence the world.

EMOTIONAL INTELLIGENCE: This Is the ability of your mind and body to maintain stability and soberly adapt to new challenges and changes. It is said that in life, change is the only constant and since the year two thousand, change has been coming at a fast and furious pace.

Emotional intelligence is the assurance of hope that enables you to be patiently confident during seasons of change even when there's no tangible indication that you will have a good outcome. This is the result of a life anchored in faith based on the knowledge of the promises of salvation that we have received in Christ.

Emotional intelligence is almost impossible to describe because it's a quality that the world would consider to be foolishness, ignorance, deception, unrealistic, out of touch with reality and such like descriptions. For example, we're told in the Bible to run with patience. How do you run while at the same time be patient? It means that your feet run while your heart maintains peace and rhythm with heaven.

*For I am not ashamed of the gospel of Christ: for it is the power of God unto salvation to every one that believeth; to the Jew first, and also to the Greek. For therein is the righteousness of God revealed from faith to faith: as it is written, **The just shall live by faith**. (Romans 1:16-17)*

Emotional Intelligence is one of the strengths of life that many lack and end up making irrational decisions that come to haunt them later. Emotional intelligence is the fruit of wisdom that saves life, weathers storms and produce success in the end. Think about all the heroes mentioned in the book of Hebrews chapter eleven and consider the

amount of emotional intelligence they needed to wage the
good fight of faith.

4. HOW TO BUILD THE PERFECT IMAGE

THE FASHION STORE OF SALVATION - *The Born Again Experience*

The greatest image problem of man is spiritual and not physical. Solving the physical image only is to apply cosmetic change that will not bring the perfect and lasting solution. The spiritual image problem can only be rectified spiritually and by none other but God.

*I will greatly rejoice in the LORD, my soul shall be joyful in my God; for he hath **clothed me with the garments of salvation**, he hath **covered me with the robe of righteousness**, as a bridegroom decketh himself with ornaments, and as a bride adorneth herself with her jewels. (Isaiah 61:10)*

The true image of man is restored when a person receives the image of Christ through salvation. This is the first and most important step in getting it right. Life is not lived in the physical plane only; life is spiritual and the spiritual is superior to the physical and controls it.

For example, if a person lacks favour, then his or her dressing, etiquette and communication skills will not come to bear. Favour is not a physical attribute but a spiritual and divine endowment upon a person that grants them access beyond their qualifications or outward packaging.

FITTING THE WARDROBE OF THE MIND – *The Transformed Mind*

The victorious life for a Christian is achieved through the supernatural power of a transformed mind. The knowledge of God is the truth that makes men free from all shackles of stagnation, confusion, persecution, sickness, lack, depression and all other limitations, obstacles, resistance and attacks from the kingdom of darkness.

The renewed mind thinks like God, understands like God, reasons like God, chooses like God and gets results like God. The renewed mind is able to discern between truth and deception, life and death and walks in the truth and wisdom of God.

And be renewed in the spirit of your mind; And that ye put on the new man, which after God is created in righteousness and true holiness. (Ephesians 4:23-24)

The benefits of the renewed mind enable a person to maintain the image of Christ from the inside out consistently and thereby receive God's virtue in the form of knowledge, soundness, boldness and a pure conscience.

For this cause we also, since the day we heard it, do not cease to pray for you, and to desire that ye might be filled with the knowledge of hls will in all wisdom and spiritual understanding; That ye might walk worthy of the Lord unto all pleasing, being fruitful in every good work, and increasing in the knowledge of God; (Colossians 1: 9-10)

The Bible says that as a man thinks so is he, meaning that our thoughts create our image that we end up projecting physically. Therefore, wrong thought will create the wrong image and the right thoughts will create the right image. We must actively engage the mind of Christ that we have received from God so that our thoughts are constantly in alignment with God's. This is what will enable us to use the shield of faith against the darts of ungodly thoughts and enticements and wield the sword of the Spirit to counter Satan's lethal suggestions and accusations.

It is in the solitary mind of man that the war between good and evil is fought and ultimately won or lost. When a person is found naked in the soul, then the enemy's darts will pierce the heart and the person will bleed to death. The whole armour of God keeps our soul secure and subsequently our image and identity.

Casting down imaginations, and every high thing that exalteth itself against the knowledge of God, and bringing into captivity every thought to the obedience of Christ; (2 Corinthians 10:5)

Without the whole armour of God, the enemy will have a field day in your soul plaguing it with fear, anger, hatred, lust, lewdness, jealousy, timidity, stifling regret, unending sorrow, hopelessness and depression. Many of the mental health conditions such as bipolar, schizophrenia, OCD, are manifestations of demonic oppression of the soul.

All these are various degrees of death which if not checked, may lead to physical sicknesses, madness, addictions, horrid violence, suicides, etc.

The Bible counsels us to be deliberate in what we allow into our minds. We daily interact with information and are involved in situations that can easily create bad thoughts in our minds. The counsel here, is to not dwell on those things. Deal with the issue at hand as soon as possible according to your ability and God's wisdom. For example, don't continue listening or watching something that will defile your thoughts. Move away, stop it if you're able to or distract yourself with something good depending on the situation.

Finally, brethren, whatsoever things are true, whatsoever things are honest, whatsoever things are pure, whatsoever things are lovely, whatsoever things are of good report; if there be any virtue, and if there be any praise, think on these things. (Philippians 4:8)

If the image and identity of a person is not secured in their mind, it doesn't matter how smartly dressed they are in the physical, they're spiritually naked and exposed to the destructive forces of darkness.

GETTING IN SHAPE THROUGH FELLOWSHIP - *Intimate walk with God*

You work on your image every day you wake up; in fact, most people have a routine of activities they do in preparation at the start of each day. No one steps outside the door without the assurance that their presentation is satisfactory, at least to themselves. The last step is to check into the mirror or ask someone to confirm that everything's okay.

Fellowship with God through prayer, studying of the word and meditation is the spiritual preparation we need before stepping out of the door each morning. However or whatever time you do it, fellowship with God is what puts you in shape to project a wholesome image throughout your day. The more of the Word of God is in us, the richer our fellowship with God will be and the more fruitful our lives will be.

Problem solving, escaping the snares of the enemy, creating new opportunities, exceeding expectations and handling other unforeseen situations require more than appearance, good behaviour and communication skills. The Holy Spirit, Jesus said, would not only remind us what we need to know for the moment, but also show us things before they happen (John 16:13). This advanced intelligence is a gamechanger for the person who engages in fellowship with God. Remember the Holy Spirit only acts on the Word and will of God.

One of the reasons why many people's images and identity are taking a beating is because they're ill equipped in their mind to accurately diagnose, interpret and prescribe the right remedy. Therefore, when they arrive at life's crossroads, thresholds and experience crisis, they get overwhelmed.

The entrance of thy words giveth light; it giveth understanding unto the simple. (Psalm 119:130)

When the Word of God richly dwells in us, we will have an accurate lens and the right intensity of light to not only interpret the real issue but also divinely source for the solution. For example, many people rely on the media to paint for them the right picture of what is transpiring in the world around them and far away.

Any believer who solely relies on the media as their primary source of news and information to guide their decision making, is cooked, and the enemy will have them for breakfast, lunch and dinner. News from the legacy media without the perspective of God's Word is to expect life from the tree of the knowledge of good and evil, an impossible feat.

It is the light of God's Word and the leadership of the Holy Spirit in us that helps us to navigate the hills and valleys, forests and plains of life as we run our course of purpose to the expected godly end. This is the only way to remain focused and steady on your path when you come across giants, ravenous wild animals, floods, wild fires, storms, deceptive detours and traps of the enemy.

For whatsoever is born of God overcometh the world: and this is the victory that overcometh the world, even our faith. (1 John 5:4)

So then faith cometh by hearing, and hearing by the word of God. (Romans 10:17)

REAPING THE BENEFITS OF GODLY IMAGE - *Exercising Godliness*

Christianity is a lifestyle and not just a mental belief, it is a practice that is exercised everyday by the believer. The constant fellowship with God is for the purpose of energizing the will to act on the Word of God through speech and action.

Godliness, the bible records is profitable in all things (1 Timothy 4:8). That means that exercising ourselves in godliness will produce fruit in our work, family, organizations, nation, and every other place of engagement. Godliness simply means to act like God, to imitate Christ. We know that Christ is perfect and therefore living like Him is to live a victorious life and we can confidently say, all things work together for our good because we love God - Romans 8:28.

Exercising godliness is to understand that ALL we do is in service to God. We may have human bosses or family to take care of and other social responsibilities but our one and true boss is God to whom we owe all accountability. He is also the one who is able to adequately reward us for our work.

And whatsoever ye do, do it heartily, as to the Lord, and not unto men; Knowing that of the Lord ye shall receive reward of the inheritance: for ye serve the Lord Christ. (Colossians 3: 23-24)

The formula for building the perfect image starts by reconnecting with God through salvation. This restores our original image and identity. Then working on our mind to bring it into alignment with the outworking of the will of God in our lives. Maintaining our connection with God through fellowship to ensure consistent and sustained reflection of the image of Christ in us and finally living out our image and identity as we explore and fulfill purpose.

5. THE LAWS GOVERNING IMAGE CONSULTANCY

THE IMPORTANCE OF LAWS

Laws are keys that God has given us to enable the realization of excellent and predictable results when we apply them. We determine what happens on earth by keys and by using the keys of the Kingdom, we can deliver heaven to the earth.

And I will give unto thee the keys of the kingdom of heaven and whatsoever thou shalt bind on earth shall be bound in heaven: and whatsoever thou shalt loose on earth shall be loosed in heaven. (Matthew 16:19)

The Word of God is what carries the knowledge of Kingdom laws or principles and therefore studying the Word and not just reading it, is what will help us to dig into the realm of understanding. The advice of God to Joshua is as relevant today as it was those many thousands of years when they were spoken to him.

This book of the law shall not depart out of thy mouth; but thou shalt meditate therein day and night, that thou mayest observe to do according to all that is written therein: for then thou shalt make thy way prosperous, and then thou shalt have good success. (Joshua 1:8)

The key to life is order and the source of order are principles. The laws of God protect, sustain, preserve, guard and promote life. The laws discussed in the following pages are applicable in other areas of life but they're specifically highlighted on how they apply to a persons' image and identity. An image consultant will have greater success by knowing how these Kingdom laws affect them and their clients.

THE LAW OF LOVE

The law of love is the foundation of image and identity. This law can be traced back to the creation of man when God decided that the template for man would be Himself. All other created things and beings were made after their own kind, but man was created in the image and likeness of God.

Man is God's most treasured creation born out of love. The love of God for man is the reason why the earth exists. It is recorded in the Bible that the earth has been given to the children of men by God. We're to rule on the earth on behalf of God, earth being an extension of heaven.

The law of love then dictates that God's image in man was given out of great love by the heavenly Father towards His children in the earth to enable them function like Him. Love compelled God to share not only His image but also His glory and honor with His children – Psalm 8:5.

Salvation itself is a story of redemptive love where Jesus steps out of heaven and humbles Himself to become like His children to suffer and die on our behalf so that we don't have to pay the penalty for our sins.

The law of love is what enables the true and divine image of a person to be restored. Without love, there's no redemption and without redemption, we're doomed with the marred image caused by the sin nature.

The love of God is the bond of perfection, it allows for the presentation of a cohesive image that's true, authentic and whole. The love of God is not self-seeking, is not easily provoked and never fails, plus many other attributes as listed in the first book of Corinthians chapter thirteen.

This love has been shed abroad in the hearts of all born again believers by the Holy Spirit (Romans 5:5) and empowers the believer to experience the virtues of God. It is love that cannot be destroyed because it is anchored not on fallible feelings or emotions but on the nature of the unchanging God, who's the same yesterday, today and forever.

Just like love compelled God to put into action the redemption plan, this law of love compels the Kingdom image consultant to desire nothing less than total restoration of the divine image and identity for their client so that the person experiences wholeness in their spirit, soul and body. The image consultant is the conduit through which God ministers life to their client.

And the very God of peace sanctify you wholly; and I pray God your whole spirit and soul and body be preserved blameless unto the coming of our Lord Jesus Christ. (1 Thessalonians 5:23)

THE LAW OF SALVATION

That if thou shalt confess with thy mouth the Lord Jesus, and shalt believe in thine heart that God hath raised him from the dead, thou shalt be saved. For with the heart man believeth unto righteousness; and with the mouth confession is made unto salvation. (Romans 10:9-10)

The fall of Adam condemned all men to fall short of the glory of God. The law of salvation demands that a person must get born again before their divine image and identity can be restored back to them. The law of salvation is fulfilled when a person accepts Jesus Christ as their Lord and Saviour which allows God to effect their transfer from the kingdom of darkness to the Kingdom of light by the regenerating power of the Holy Spirit.

Therefore if any man be in Christ, he is a new creature: old things are passed away; behold, all things are become new. (2 Corinthians 5:17)

I still remember vividly the day I gave my life to Christ. I had reached the end of my road and had lost all hope for the future. Having come from a broken family where life was full of uncertainties and constant wrangles, I was two years out after finishing High School and I didn't see a clear path into my future. I was on my own and the task of achieving my life dreams seemed impossible.

A dark and heavy cloud of hopelessness settled firmly on my shoulders and threatened to blind me and also bury me. It was at that point that I cried out to God for help and committed my life to Him. The change and relief was instant; the dark cloud disappeared, my heart swelled with joy and peace I had never felt before in my life. The tears of sadness changed to tears of joy and my outlook of life changed for good.

The law of salvation redeems a person from eternal damnation and darkness to eternal life, hope and life in abundance. The Kingdom image consultant works with God to reconcile those who are not saved and lead them back to God in order to receive their divine image and identity. The image consultant also works with believers who need help in packaging and expressing their image and identity.

THE LAW OF THE SPIRIT OF LIFE

The law of the Spirit of life is the law of daily living a life empowered by the Word and the Spirit of God. This law is the most important one in image consultancy because it maintains the original and perfect image as God envisioned for man in the beginning (Genesis 1:26-27). It is the law of daily victorious living because it helps the believer to operate above the vagaries of the world system.

The term law does not refer primarily to any written code, but mainly to authority or power. The law of the Spirit is the authority and power of the Spirit and the return you get is sanctification whose end is eternal life. As many as are led by the Spirit of God, these are the sons of God. These are the ones from whom condemnation has been removed.

The spirit of a man is quickened (made alive) when the Holy Spirit comes to indwell the spirit of the person and this act confers a higher authority and supernatural power to overcome the previous enslaving power of sin in the flesh. Without the power of the Holy Spirit, no man can overcome the weakness of the flesh and the sin virus that works in it.

For the law of the Spirit of life in Christ Jesus hath made me free from the law of sin and death. (Romans 8:2)

The person who is not born again cannot experience the full expression of their image because appearance, behaviour and communication are perfected in Christ alone. Anything outside of Christ does not carry the full import of divine potential and purpose. The law of the Spirit of life in Christ Jesus allows for the full and total expression of the Christ man, the perfect image and identity.

THE LAW OF SIN AND DEATH

The law of sin and death was activated when man fell and from that moment death began to reign through sin. Everything governed by the law of sin and death tends to death. Everything governed by this law decreases in value and quality with successive use/reproduction or as time elapses. That's why the world and everything in it is not getting better. The technological advancements being hailed currently are but breeding grounds for bigger compounded problems in the future.

For all have sinned, and come short of the glory of God. (Romans 3:23)

Wherefore, as by one man sin entered into the world, and death by sin; and so death passed upon all men, for that all have sinned: (Romans 5:12)

Any civilization that man builds apart from God has no long-term value and definitely no eternal value. That's why the Bible records that all of creation is groaning and awaiting salvation (Romans 8:19-21). The law of sin and death is the root cause of the image malfunction experienced by men.

For as long as a person is not born again, they're without choice subject to the law of sin and death. This law works to produce all the crossroads, thresholds and predicaments of life that impair the image of a person. The operation of this law has to be stopped and nullified in order to experience the fulness of man's image as written in God's book for every individual. That's why the Kingdom image consultant should be able to tell if a client needs the law of salvation to be activated in their client's life.

That as sin hath reigned unto death, even so might grace reign through righteousness unto eternal life by Jesus Christ our Lord. (Romans 5:21)

THE LAW OF THE TRANSFORMED MIND

The mind of Christ operates at God level where it becomes possible to know the thoughts and ways of God. This was the difference between Moses and the children of Israel. The transformed mind is the launch pad for doing exploits, fulfilling purpose and actualization in life.

For who hath known the mind of the Lord, that he may instruct him? But we have the mind of Christ. (1 Corinthians 2:16)

Many people though, struggle with their image because the world has succeeded to infect their minds with the mental virus called carnality. The children of Israel at the brink of entering into the promised land squandered the moment by allowing fear to infect their mind. In their own minds, they pictured themselves to be as grasshoppers. This is despite the fact that God had made their enemies to be like bread to them. Just like that, they forfeited their inheritance with a forty-year delay until all the adults of that generation died except for Joshua and Caleb.

Many people make the same mistake as the children of Israel everyday by viewing their lives through the lenses of the world (the happenings in their surroundings and life experiences) instead of the Word of God. The giants in the world look terrible and impossible to defeat, that's why the Bible trains our mind to focus on heaven's technology, techniques and resources to overcome the world.

Since, then, you have been raised with Christ, set your hearts on things above, where Christ is, seated at the right hand of God. Set your minds on things above, not on earthly things. For you died, and your life is now hidden with Christ in God. (Colossians 3:1-3 NIV)

For to be carnally minded is death; but to be spiritually minded is life and peace. (Romans 8:6)

The world wants you to focus on survival mentality, on conniving your way out of the pressures and hard situations of life. The shortcuts of the world look easier and faster in order to get desired results but the longest route to success is a shortcut. Righteousness is no longer attractive in the world but viewed as old fashioned and upholding it is being judgmental on others or even infringing on other people's rights. In the end though, the way of a carnal mind leads to death and destruction.

The law of the transformed mind keeps the person in perfect peace irrespective of the storms of life because there's an understanding and assurance that greater is He that is on the inside than the one on the outside. God also keeps him or her in perfect peace whose mind is stayed on Him – Isaiah 26:3.

THE LAW OF THE FRUIT OF THE LIPS

The law of the fruit of the lips is governed by God's wisdom and understanding and directs the lips to give the right communication for every occasion. The lips represent the mouth's ability to produce sound in form of audible words that carry meaning originating from the heart.

The lips are the communication medium that open or lock doors of opportunity for a person. The lips connected to a heart full of God's wisdom and understanding is a wellspring of life that goes beyond the ability to structure good sentences but also deliver divine insight and sound instruction.

The righteous person invests time in the Word and in fellowship with God to acquire the wisdom that comes from above which is pure, peaceable, gentle, easy to entreat, full of mercy and good fruits, without partiality, and without hypocrisy - James 3:17.

Let's sample a few benefits from the Bible book of Proverbs how the lips of a righteous man preserve his life, delivers him from destruction, earns him respect and favour and so much more.

Bring success: *A man's belly shall be satisfied with the fruit of his mouth; and with the increase of his lips shall he be filled. (Proverbs 18:20)*

Bring favour: *Righteous lips are the delight of kings; and they love him that speaketh right. (Proverbs 16:13)*

Add knowledge: *The heart of the wise teacheth his mouth, and addeth learning to his lips. (Proverbs 16:23)*

Does not speak impulsively: *Even a fool, when he holdeth his peace, is counted wise: and he that shutteth his lips is esteemed a man of understanding. (Proverbs 17:28)*

Teach others the right way: *The lips of the wise disperse knowledge: but the heart of the foolish doeth not so. (Proverbs 15: 7)*

A resource of knowledge: *That thou mayest regard discretion, and that thy lips may keep knowledge. (Proverbs 5:2)*

Treasures and holds truth: *For my mouth shall speak truth; and wickedness is an abomination to my lips. (Proverbs 8:7)*

Helps other people: *The lips of the righteous feed many: but fools die for want of wisdom. (Proverbs 10:21)*

Is acquainted with what is right: *The lips of the righteous know what is acceptable: but the mouth of the wicked speaketh forwardness. (Proverbs 10:32)*

Keeps you from ensnaring yourself: *A fool's mouth is his destruction, and his lips are the snare of his soul. (Proverbs 18:7)*

Keeps you from deception: *Be not a witness against thy neighbour without cause; and deceive not with thy lips. (Proverbs 24:28)*

Keeps you from self-promotion and thinking of yourself more highly than you ought: *Let another man praise thee, and not thine own mouth; a stranger and not thine own lips. (Proverbs 27:2)*

The law of the fruit of the lips teaches a person behavioral and communication skill that are able to open new doors of opportunities and build great relationships that can be leveraged to obtain good outcomes for the individual, family, business, organization, community, nation or for global good.

The Kingdom image consultant understands that it's out of the abundance of the heart that the mouth speaks and therefore focuses on getting the heart right in order to the get the speech right. Things like pride, deceit, lust, envy, jealousy can contaminate the heart. Putting in just a temporary effort to change vocabulary in order to achieve a certain outcome will soon be reversed when the task is achieved or discarded. The Kingdom image consultant should not work with a client just for short term gain.

THE LAW OF PURPOSE

"Before I formed you in the womb I knew you, before you were born I set you apart; I appointed you as a prophet to the nations." (Jeremiah 1:5 NIV)

The law of purpose should be a source of great hope for any person especially those who may consider themselves not to have been born under ideal circumstances or on the right side of the tracks. It doesn't matter how or where you were born, all that is subject to change and to align with the purpose of God as predetermined before your conception.

The quoted scripture above reveals to us a critical truth; our origin is in God and therefore as our source, He is also our sustainer. We're not to try and figure out how we're to survive or thrive in this crazy world, all we have to find out is the content of the divine script as written by God in our individual image and identity book.

A script lets you know how the entire story will play out before the first character steps on the scene. God has not left our lives to chance, He planned out each day of our lives and the purpose we're to ultimately accomplish. King David discovered this knowledge and prayed to God to teach him to number his days – Psalm 39:4.

Knowledge of your purpose gives strength to endure the tough seasons because you know it's just a phase and not the end. This knowledge is what made Joseph not to compromise or to give up hope when things seemed to go off script. In our journey of purpose, the enemy of our soul will seek to find every opportunity to derail us. We must firmly be rooted in our conviction of our divine predestination, lest we buy into his lies and trickery.

In whom also we have obtained an inheritance, being predestinated according to the purpose of him who worketh all things after the counsel of his own will: (Ephesians 1:11)

Our knowledge and trust in God will be tested by fiery trials but we're told that these only act as catalysts for refining our faith which is much more precious than gold. When trouble comes, we look unto Jesus, who is the author and finisher of our faith. He is the rock upon which we're founded and no storm can uproot us from there. Knowledge of the divine purpose and the outworking of God in us to fulfill that purpose generates a much stronger force and power than all the power of the kingdom of darkness.

But we have this treasure in earthen vessels, that the excellency of the power may be of God, and not of us. We are troubled on every side, yet not distressed; we are perplexed, but not in despair; Persecuted, but not forsaken; cast down, but not destroyed; (2 Corinthians 4: 7-9)

It is impossible for the child of God to not fulfill purpose. It is impossible because, it is God who is at work in us both to will and to do (Philippians 2:13) and He never fails. No one who ever trusted in God's plan and faithfulness experienced abortion of purpose no matter the trials they went through. This was the testimony of Noah, Abraham, Joseph, Moses, David, Daniel and his three friends, the Apostles and disciples of the early church. It is the same God who honoured their faith that is now at work in us. Satan has no chance of winning against you.

The only condition is that we remain steadfast in our faith in God and in the knowledge of His good purpose for our lives. Pursue the Kingdom first and God's righteousness as you walk in your path of righteousness as the Holy Spirit leads. The Kingdom image consultant works to help their client articulate their God given purpose in order to gain clarity and direction.

THE LAW OF CONSECRATION AND ABIDING

The law of consecration dictates that we're set apart for God's use only. Having been bought at a price, we no longer live for ourselves, we live to please our Lord and saviour and His will we seek to do at all times. True freedom is found by the child of God who surrenders his or her life to the leading and guidance of God.

Lord means owner and if Jesus is your Lord, then your life has to be lived according to His will. Many Christians live their lives with God simply acting as a rubberstamp for their plans, desires and wishes. As human beings we're limited in our ability to know what the future portends. That's why the Bible counsels that we should not lean on our own understanding and to remember to acknowledge God in all our ways so that He may direct our paths – Proverbs 3:5-6.

It is our responsibility to choose to become vessels of honour in God's house for His use. The consecrated life is devoid of worldly pollution. The Holy Spirit empowers you to live a pure life in the midst of a perverse and wicked generation. This was the secret of Daniel and his three friends who lived victoriously in Babylon. As the world becomes darker and darker, living a consecrated life is how we will escape the corruption that's in it.

According as his divine power hath given unto us all things that pertain unto life and godliness, through the knowledge of him that hath called us to glory and virtue: Whereby are given unto us exceeding great and precious promises: that by these ye might be partakers of the divine nature, having escaped the corruption that is in the world through lust. (2Peter 1: 3-4)

Consecration and abiding enable the believer to be in tune with heaven and the Holy Spirit at all times. This is the place where the enemy is locked out by the firewall of the Holy Spirit and none of his virus can infect the mind to cause a malfunction of God's image and divine identity given to you.

While consecration keeps you intact from worldly pollution, abiding is the place of producing the power to change the world. Jesus told us that if we abide in Him and Him in us, then we will produce fruit – John 15:1-11. Abiding is the place of fellowship with God and beholding Jesus in the Word until we're transformed into His image from glory to glory.

Abiding is you drawing from the life of Christ and living it out as you project that image and identity which is Christ in you through your speech and actions. Abiding is one of the important keys that unlock good success in the life of a believer. This is how you get to work and not toil, work that brings you fulfillment and reward for the life that now is and the one to come.

If you abide in Me, and My words abide in you, you will ask what you desire, and it shall be done for you. By this My Father is glorified, that you bear much fruit; so you will be My disciples. (John 15:7-8 NIV)

THE LAW OF NAMES AND NAMING

What's in a name? Well, a name carries personality, power and authority. That's why in Christianity, the name given to a person is of vital interest. We find in the Bible irrefutable evidence of consequences of right or bad naming. There are also several instances when God intervened and changed the names of people which did not align with His will for those particular individuals. Such was the case for Abraham and Jacob.

Personality encapsulates the character of a person, power refers to the gifts and talents, the graces upon an individual's life and authority is the right to use the giftings and calling to accomplish purpose. A name therefore is the declaration of who a person is in a nutshell. A name is the audible version of your image and identity.

There are various ways we acquire names and it's critical that we take note of the sources from which we're named. The first place where we acquire our name is from our parents. Based on their level of knowledge or insight into

God's working, parents give good, neutral or bad names to their children. Neutral names are those that have no meaning, they're often chosen because of the way they sound.

The other way in which somebody can acquire a name is when other people out of interaction or observation, decide to give a new or secondary name to someone. This happens to people who are good in a particular activity like sports, skill, etc. It can also be given due to certain physical features that stand out in a person. Some nicknames are good while others are for ridicule or given due to a bad reputation. A good example is when Jesus gave Simon a new name, "Peter" which means "a mass of rock detached from the living rock."

The third way people acquire names is by self-naming according to how they view themselves in their mind. This can have an empowering effect or create a negative and defeating self-image. The name you give to yourself can act as a catalyst that propels you towards your God ordained destiny or it can become the stumbling block that brings you to a halt. You should name yourself according to the revelation you receive in God's Word in line with your purpose. It is good to call yourself by the names that God calls us in His Word. For example, you can call yourself a king, more than a conqueror, son of God, ambassador, etc.

The law of naming demands that you accept only the names that are in alignment with God's will. Any other name that does not align must be dropped like a hot potato because it will cause a conflict with your image and identity. By faith we understand that the worlds were framed by the Word of God meaning that words carry potent power. Therefore, let the power that is released every time your name is called be one that declare your greatness, success, destiny, potential, divine attribute or purpose.

For to us a child is born, to us a son is given, and the government will be on his shoulders. And he will be called Wonderful Counselor, Mighty God, Everlasting Father, Prince of Peace. (Isaiah 9:6 NIV)

THE LAW OF SACRIFICE

Sacrificial living is one of the hallmarks of Christianity. Our bodies are to be offered as holy and living sacrifice and our lifestyle should mirror that of a soldier. Sacrificial living is important because we have an adversary who although already defeated, still masquerades as a lion seeking whom he may devour. Our part is not to defeat him but to resist him. Jesus already defeated Satan through His shed blood.

The law of sacrifice helps us to stay grounded and not to think of ourselves more highly than we ought to. Our strengths if not checked can also be the source of our weakness which the enemy can easily exploit to our downfall. Someone who is excellent at a particular skill or knowledge can easily be infected with pride. Physical beauty can deceive a lady into thinking they're superior to others. Wealth can deceive someone into thinking they're invincible and take lightly their dependency on God.

And that which fell among thorns are they, which, when they have heard, go forth, and are chocked with cares and riches and pleasures of this life, and bring no fruit to perfection. (Luke 8:14)

The law of sacrifice is what keeps you from going overboard or into excesses of life due to spiritual endowment or natural resources in your possession. Realizing that you're a small part in the grand scheme of the Kingdom makes you run your race with temperance knowing that this race started a long time ago and that it's now your awesome privilege to carry the baton, run diligently according to the rules and handover to the next generation.

A sacrificial life is not self-absorbed, it seeks for the common good of everyone and delights in co-labouring with God in the ministry of reconciliation. Your image and identity are given to enable you effectively serve others. It's not for looking cute and boasting about your resources, abilities and features.

You therefore must endure hardship as a good soldier of Jesus Christ. (2 Timothy 2:3 NKJV)

THE LAW OF ETERNITY

Yet God has made everything beautiful for its own time. He has planted eternity in the human heart, but even so, people cannot see the whole scope of God's work from beginning to end. (Ecclesiastes 3:11 NLT)

Life on earth is a short time compared to eternity, we therefore ought to live with our eyes set on the life after here. We can't afford to live life focused only on the things that happen within time on earth, that is to be shortsighted.

Eternity is the real deal and with that in mind, we live our lives on earth in a way that will secure the best position for us in eternity. Any sacrifice made on earth is too small for the reward we will receive and enjoy in eternity.

For our light affliction, which is but for a moment, is working for us a far more exceeding and eternal weight of glory, (2 Corinthians 4:17 NKJV)

If you understand this reality then you'll appreciate why some of the heroes of faith mentioned in the eleventh chapter of Hebrews refused to be spared of their lives but chose, rather to die because they did not count their lives on earth dear unto themselves. They considered their faith in God more valuable than life without acknowledging the existence of the almighty God.

The law of eternity will help you to pay the price so that no matter the affliction the enemy may subject you too, you'll not in your own strength or ingenuity try to save yourself, but will rather choose the truth and the will of God whether it leads to exploits of stopping the mouth of lions or death.

David before he became king had the perfect opportunity to eliminate king Saul and ascend to the throne as he had already been anointed as king over Israel by Prophet Samuel, but he chose not to do it his way but wait for God's time. David later on testified that indeed it was God who elevated him to the throne.

So David knew that the LORD had established him as king over Israel, and that He had exalted His kingdom for the sake of His people Israel. (2 Samuel 5:12 NKJV)

Until, you can declare like Apostle Paul said in the scripture below, the enemy will be able to exploit your fears and force you to compromise on your values.

For to me to live is Christ, and to die is gain. (Philippians 1:21)

The fear of death has held many Christians into bondage and they find themselves responding to the impulses of the enemy instead of by faith in God. Death produces the greatest fear in men and that's one of the snares that Jesus Christ dealt with on the cross. The Bible tells us that we have not received the spirit of fear, but of power, of love and of a sound mind (2 Timothy 1:7).

Perfect love casts out fear (1 John 4:18) and this awesome love of God is also the bond of perfection (Colossians 3:14). If you therefore find your heart being plagued by crippling fear of the known or unknown, just ask God to perfect you in His love. The love of God is a much greater power than death, that's why the grave couldn't hold on to Jesus. The love of God is life and life in abundance, choose love, receive life and victory.

Forasmuch then as the children are partakers of flesh and blood, he also himself likewise took part of the same; that through death he might destroy him that had the power of death, that is, the devil; And deliver them who through fear of death were all their lifetime subject to bondage. (Hebrews 2:14-15)

The law of eternity grants you the heavenly perspective of life on earth and the bigger picture of the culmination of all matters. With this in mind, our confidence is not in our own abilities but in the power of God that is at work in us. It is through this power that we're able to receive and enjoy the exceeding and abundant supply from heaven that is above what we can ask or think (Ephesians 3:20).

THE LAW OF DOMINION

And God blessed them, and God said unto them, Be fruitful, and multiply, and replenish the earth, and subdue it: and have dominion over the fish of the sea, and over the fowl of the air, and over every living thing that moveth upon the earth. (Genesis 1:28)

Every individual human being is divinely wired to have dominion in a particular area of life. Having dominion is not just a command that God gave to Adam and Eve in the beginning but an ability that God gave to man in order to take care of the earth.

This means that everybody is equipped with certain abilities that when harnessed into skill through knowledge, understanding and wisdom will make a person fruitful in their work and grow to the place of dominion. Your image and identity are part of this divine equipping as it embodies the expression of all your abilities and potential.

The law of dominion helps you to know that you have inherent value and power to change or overcome limiting forces until you come to the place of dominion. Dominion is not a preserve of a few, it is the destiny of every human being and it's best achieved in and through God. Your image and identity is not subject to change by circumstances, it is circumstances that are to change and align with the predestined blueprint of your life.

We have an assurance from God that the position of those who have received Jesus Christ as their Lord and saviour are to be rulers in this present life. To rule over circumstances, nature, forces, dominate principles and accomplish purpose.

For if by one man's offence death reigned by one; much more they which receive abundance of grace and of the gift of righteousness shall reign in life by one, Jesus Christ. (Romans 5:17)

We have been given authority and power over all the power of Satan. Whatever we bind on earth is bound in heaven and whatever we loose on earth is loosed in heaven. We're not at the mercy of evil forces, we're in charge of our lives, families, communities and nations.

And he said unto them, Go ye into all the world, and preach the gospel to every creature. He that believeth and is baptized shall be saved; but he that believeth not shall be damned. And these signs shall follow them that believe; In my name shall they cast out devils; they shall speak with new tongues; They shall take up serpents; and if they drink any deadly thing, it shall not hurt them; they shall lay hands on the sick, and they shall recover. (Mark 16:15-18)

The purpose of your image and identity is to exercise dominion. Maximize its full potential now. Don't hold back and don't fear.

THE LAW OF SUBSTITUTION AND ACCESS

I am crucified with Christ: nevertheless I live; yet not I, but Christ liveth in me: and the life which I now live in the flesh I live by the faith of the Son of God, who loved me, and gave himself for me. (Galatians 2:20)

Another reason why people struggle with their image and identity is because it's tough work to keep up with the demands of the world. The standards of the world keep shifting like the length of shadows from sunrise to sunset. It is so by design because the world system is not meant to help you succeed but to make you a miserable failure.

By the world standards shall no man experience their true image and identity. You will never be good enough in the world for or at anything. The world uses people and then dumps them and pick up new people to use and this cycle of use and dump operates in a perpetual loop. The only way to truly thrive and reach full potential is by substituting your life for that of Christ.

For He made Him who knew no sin to be sin for us, that we might become the righteousness of God in Him. (2 Corinthians 5:21)

It is not enough to just get saved. Getting saved brings you into the Kingdom but in order to enjoy the possibilities, you must be prepared to engage further. The purpose of the substitution is to grant you unfettered access to the throne of God where you can directly obtain mercy and grace and every resource of heaven you need.

You make use of the access by making a conscious decision to let Christ live in and through you. Putting on clothes is a conscious decision where you choose which one to wear at a given time or occasion. It takes thought, consideration and action to dress up. Similarly, every day, we must make the decision to let Christ be the one that lives through us.

Rather, clothe yourselves with the Lord Jesus Christ, and do not think about how to gratify the desires of the flesh. (Romans 13:14 NIV)

Christ is perfect, He is the same, yesterday, today and forever. Christ is consistent, right, able, reliable, unfailing, true, and everything else that is good and perfect. The person who chooses to let Christ reign in their lives will never experience image meltdowns or identity crisis.

THE LAW OF PERCEPTION

According to the Oxford English Dictionary, perception is the process of becoming aware or conscious of a thing or things in general; the state of being aware; consciousness; understanding.

According to an article by the University of Chicago on Theories of Media, the word perception refers to what the body is able to perceive, that is, the information that the body is able to discern from the outside world.

The process of understanding becomes a mediated experience, as it requires the use of the senses in order to process data. To be perceivable, the object must be able to be understood by the mind through the interplay of sight, sound, taste, touch and smell. To be perceived, a sensation must pass through the body through one of the sensory organs, that is, the eye, ear, nose, mouth, or skin. To interpret that sensation is what is known as perception. The perceivable is that which can be interpreted by the body.

Our focus though is on spiritual perception. Perception that is limited to interpretation based on the physical senses alone is not sufficient to discern spiritual movements. We're spiritual beings and the ability to perceive what's going on in the spiritual realm is not an option for the child of God.

Since you have been raised to new life with Christ, set your sights on the realities of heaven, where Christ sits in the place of honor at God's right hand. (Colossians 3:1 NLT)

In order to get the right and true perspective of everything that is happening on the earth, you must know the position of heaven. Only the position of heaven captures the original intent (beginning) and the future (conclusion) of a matter. With this knowledge, you can accurately judge what's happening currently because in the spiritual realm there's no limitation of knowledge. No one can pretend or masquerade in that realm and if you operate from there, you can never be deceived or lied to.

Many people have suffered loss and pain because they did not check with heaven to find out God's position on a matter. Assumption is the lowest level of knowledge and a good example is when the children of Israel were tricked into a covenant by the Gibeonites. Joshua, the priests and the elders did not enquire from God but made a decision based on what they had perceived by their natural senses.

One of the best ways to increase your level of spiritual perception is by praying in the spirit. According to Romans 8:26, we suffer limitation in the place of prayer because we don't know the will of God, but the Holy Spirit knows. Therefore, He is able to accurately intercede on our behalf before the Father. Praying in the spirit is to offer perfect prayers that the Father takes pleasure in answering.

Christians continue to be deceived into relationships that break and wound their hearts, business deals that defraud them of their finances, traps that lead them into sin and compromise. These things ought not to be so.

If you need to make a decision and you don't have full information, take time and pray in the spirit. Any time you feel challenged in a particular area, spend time praying in the spirit until you perceive the answer or solution.

And the Father who knows all hearts knows what the Spirit is saying, for the Spirit pleads for us believers in harmony with God's own will. (Romans 8:27 NLT)

CONCLUSION

Our God given image and identity is what enables us to have dominion on the earth and to fulfill our purpose. This image and identity is the greatest threat to Satan and his kingdom. He managed to destroy it for a season when Adam and Eve believed his lies. Jesus has restored it back to everyone who accepts salvation.

Our part is to guard it by holding on to truth, living out the truth and helping others to find out the truth. We're all image consultants in one way or the other. You may specialize on it as a professional and help many people, or you may simply influence those within your environment to embrace God's blueprint for their lives.

The greatest pandemic of our time is the one affecting mental health. Satan knows that if he captures the minds of men, then he can control them into his desired outcome. We have the truth that is able to make men free, let's be the light in an increasing dark world.

THE ROLE OF FASHION

Fashion is about expressing our divine identity and aiding us in fulfilling purpose through appropriate spiritual, mental and physical fitting. The primary function of fashion therefore, is the equipping for purpose. To picture this more clearly, we can ask ourselves the following question.

Can the lion fulfill purpose without its fashion? Can the Peacock be a Peacock without its fashion? Purpose is serving and executing the will of God in accordance to His will and righteousness.

Therefore, fashion is about the establishment of the Kingdom of God on earth as it is in heaven. Fashion is a medium through which the Kingdom of God finds a radiant, diverse and colourful expression on the earth.

Fashion is a medium through which the gospel of the Kingdom of God is delivered to men and all creation as captured in Psalm 19:1-6. Fashion is the implementation of the ministry of reconciliation and the restoration of the image and likeness of God in men.

When a person gets healed, delivered from demonic oppression, raised from the dead, or gets saved, it is their fashion restored. The mistake we make sometimes is we think of fashion in terms of clothes and accessories while God thinks of fashion in terms of purpose and identity.

Fashion is the progressive expression and fulfillment of God's idea (purpose and identity) from the spirit, soul and body of a person.

The full and total expression of fashion is the fulfillment of purpose. The fulfillment of purpose is to become like Christ in your area of calling. Therefore, the true essence of fashion is to become like Christ.

Fashion is Christlikeness. That's why at the end of it all, we shall all be changed into His image and be like Him in all respect. Therefore, fashion is not about clothes, fashion is about Christ in you.

But we all, with unveiled face, beholding as in a mirror the glory of the Lord, are being transformed into the same image from glory to glory, just as by the Spirit of the Lord. (2 Corinthians 3:18 NKJV)

The image of God and the divine identity that we receive comes from the Kingdom which cannot be shaken. When things fall apart in the world and around you, your image and identity will prevail.

And this word, Yet once more, signifieth the removing of those things that are shaken, as of things that are shaken, as of things that are made, that those things which cannot be shaken may remain. Wherefore we receiving a kingdom which cannot be moved, let us have grace, whereby we may serve God acceptably with reverence and godly fear: (Hebrews 12:27-28)

Wear who you're, put on Christ.

#TheKingIsComing

#ImageIsEverything

ABOUT KINGDOM FASHION

Kingdom Fashion is an organization that works with Christians called into the fashion industry. The primary aim of the organization is to create an enabling environment and eco system where professionals in this industry can do fashion like God.

The secondary aim which is closely tied to the first one is to reconcile the world of fashion back to God by influencing peoples' mindset and culture through fashion. Fashion is a powerful medium for influencing everyday lifestyle in all its diverse settings.

These two primary goals are achieved through development of relevant literature, organizing training workshops, skills transfer, business incubation and launching, networking and fellowship.

Go ye therefore, and teach all nations, baptizing them in the name of the Father, and of the Son, and of the Holy Ghost: Teaching them to observe all things whatsoever I have commanded you: and, lo, I am with you always, even unto the end of the world. Amen. (Matthew 28: 19-20)

THE KINGDOM IMAGE CONSULTANT

A publication of Kingdom Fashion, Copyright ©2022.

info@kingdomfashion.co.ke

www.kingdomfashion.co.ke

Other Book Titles

- God The Fashion Designer
- The Business of Kingdom Fashion
- My Dress My Choice

www.ingramcontent.com/pod-product-compliance
Lightning Source LLC
Chambersburg PA
CBHW060111260726
48658CB00004B/1503